Cooking to Heal™

Nutrition and Cooking Class
For autism and special diets

Nutrition and Diet

Nutrient Density

Quality Foods

Soaking and Fermenting Seeds

Desserts

Fermented Foods

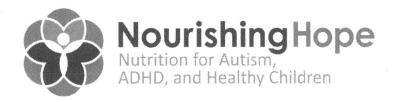

Nourishing Hope
Nutrition for Autism,
ADHD, and Healthy Children

Reading this Book

Recipes are labeled to make it easier to find the recipes you want and that are compliant with a diet you are following. In some cases, a recipe can be made compliant with a particular substitution – and is labeled, for example, as LOD, and the LOD modification is mentioned in the beginning notes of the recipe. Be sure to read the full recipe in order to make it compliant to your specific recipe needs.

The diets are marked as:

Gluten-free and Casein-free (and Soy-Free) (GFCF)
Specific Carbohydrate Diet or GAPS Diet (SCD/Gaps)
Paleo Diet (Paleo)
Low Oxalate Diet (LOD)
Body Ecology Diet (BED)
Feingold Diet (FG)
Failsafe Diet (FS)

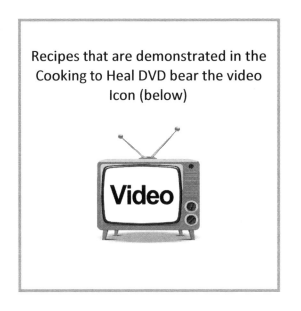

Recipes that are demonstrated in the Cooking to Heal DVD bear the video Icon (below)

There are many people who are egg-free and nut-free so I have marked these recipes as well. You will want to confirm your sources and ensure there is no cross-contamination for highly sensitive people.

Egg-Free: These recipes are egg-free or can be made that way. Read all of the instructions on each recipe for egg substitutes.

Nut-Free: These recipes are peanut-free and tree nut-free, or can be made that way. These recipes may contain seeds or coconut. If these ingredients are also not tolerated, avoid or adapt these recipes accordingly. It does not include coconut-free. Read all of the instructions on each recipe.

GFCF and Soy-Free: Everything is this cookbook is **gluten-free, casein-free, and soy-free** – with the exception of a few recipes in the Fermented Foods section that are well marked as containing dairy. For short, I refer to these recipes as "GFCF," but note that they are also soy-free.

Make sure all of your ingredients and spices are gluten-free and allergen-free.

Conversion Charts

Volume Conversions: Liquids

US Quantity	Metric Equivalent – milliliters
1 teaspoon	5 mL
1 tablespoon *or* 1/2 fluid ounce	15 mL
1 fluid ounce *or* 1/8 cup	30 mL
1/4 cup *or* 2 fluid ounces	60 mL
1/3 cup	80 mL
1/2 cup *or* 4 fluid ounces	120 mL
2/3 cup	160 mL
3/4 cup *or* 6 fluid ounces	180 mL
1 cup *or* 8 fluid ounces *or* half a pint	240 mL
1 1/2 cups *or* 12 fluid ounces	350 mL
2 cups *or* 1 pint *or* 16 fluid ounces	475 mL
3 cups *or* 1 1/2 pints	700 mL
4 cups *or* 2 pints *or* 1 quart	950 mL
4 quarts *or* 1 gallon	3.8 L

Weight Conversions

US Quantity	Metric equivalent - grams
1 ounce	28 g
4 ounces *or* 1/4 pound	113 g
8 ounces *or* 1/2 pound	230 g
2/3 pound	300 g
12 ounces *or* 3/4 pound	340 g
1 pound *or* 16 ounces	450 g
2 pounds	900 g

Weights of common ingredients

Ingredient	1 cup	1 Tbsp
Flour, grain	120 g	8 g
Sugar, granulated cane	200 g	8 g
Rice, grain uncooked	190 g	12 g
Salt	300 g	20 g
Coconut oil	220 g	14 g
Nuts, chopped	150 g	10 g
Nuts, ground	120 g	8 g

Table of Contents

Nutrition and Diet

Why Special Diets? 1

Digestion Connection 2

Gluten-Free and Casein-Free (GFCF) Cooking 6

GFCF Implementation Steps 8

Specific Carbohydrate Diet (SCD) 9

& Gut and Psychology Syndrome (GAPS) Diet..9

Food Substances...12

Meal Planning...16

Meal Ideas 17

Tools of the Trade 19

Eggs and Egg Substitutes 20

 Egg Replacer by Ener-G Foods 20

 No Egg by Orgran 20

 Baking Soda and Water 20

 Flax Seed and Water (Flax Seeds Are Not SCD Compliant)..............................21

 Pureed Fruit or Vegetable 21

 Gelatin 21

 Arrowroot Powder 21

Nutrient Density

Stocks and Broths...23

 Chicken Stock 24

 Veggie Stock 24

 Acorn or Butternut Squash Soup 25

 Stew...25

 SCD Stew 26

Kid-Friendly Vegetables..27

 Sneaking Nutrients in the Diet 27

 Making Purees 29

 Mashed Cauliflower "Potatoes" 29

 Cauliflower Rice...29

 Roasted Cauliflower 30

 Kale Chips 30

 Brussels Sprouts Chips...31

 Zucchini Chips 31

 Carrot Chips 32

 Carrot Fries 32

 Winter Squash French Fries 33

 Butternut Hash Browns 33

 Squash Pancakes 33

 Banana Pancakes 34

 Confetti Brussels Sprouts 34

 Green Beans and Almonds 35

 Broccoli with Lemon and Sesame Seeds 35

 Vegetable Latkes 36

 Potato and Vegetable Latkes..36

Beet Herb Salad with Pomegranate 37

Kale Salad 37

Juicing...39

The Beginner Juice...40

Enzymes Juice...40

Digestion Juice...40

Potassium...40

Iron...40

Anti-Inflammatory..40

Antioxidants..40

Smoothies...41

Green Smoothie..41

Quality Foods

Pasture-Raised Animal Foods and Fats 43

Squash Meatballs 44

Vegetable Meat Patties...45

Chicken Nuggets..45

Egg-Free Chicken Nuggets...46

Chicken Pancakes...46

Egg-Free Chicken Pancakes..47

Burgers with Liver...47

Chicken Sticks or Cakes..48

Egg-Free Chicken Patties...49

Stir Fry Without Soy Sauce...49

Pot Roast (Dutch oven)...50

Salmon Cakes...50

Salmon Burgers...51

Frittata Singles...51

Deviled Eggs...52

Soaking Seeds & Grains..**56**

Enzyme-rich Foods: 54

Milks & Butters..56

Nut Milk 56

Cashew Milk..56

Seed Milk..57

Coconut Milk – Dried Coconut...57

Cashew Cream...57

Hemp Cream...58

Coconut Whipped Cream..58

Rice/Oat Milk..59

Crispy Almonds...59

Crispy Nuts..60

Crispy Seeds...60

Roasted Pumpkin Seeds..60

Snack Mix..61

Nut Butter...61

Soaked Bean Dishes...62

Yellow Lentil Pancakes (Moong Dal Chila)..62

Dosas (Fermented Lentil/Rice Pancakes)..62

Roasted Garbanzo Bean Snack 63

Bean Burgers 64

LOD Bean Burgers..65

Egg-Free Bean Burgers with Rice 65

Boston Baked Beans 66

Garbanzo and Squash Stew 67

Grain-Free Bread/Baking...68

Light White Bread – 1 Loaf 68

Cashew Butter Bread 68

Nut Butter Pancake 69

Coconut Pancakes (Grain-Free) 69

Banana Pancakes (with Coconut Flour Blend) 70

Grain-Free Herb Crackers 70

Grain-Free Cereal 71

Cashew Butter Tortillas 71

Banana-Coconut Bread 71

Crispy Chickpea Flour Pancakes 72

Chickpea Pancakes 73

Gluten-Free Grain Recipes...74

Julie and Carla's Granola 74

LOD Pancakes Without Eggs 75

Breads From Anna™ - Yeast-Free Bread Mix 75

Unleavened Indian Bread (Chapati) 76

Rice Porridge (Slow Cooker) 76

Desserts

Coconut Date Balls 79

Chocolate Chip "Raw Cookie Dough" Balls...79

Coconut White Fudge 80

Cocoa Mints...80

Chocolate (Avocado) Pudding 81

Sunflower Butter Brownies 81

Chocolate Chip Cookies 82

Oat Flour Chocolate Chip Cookies 82

Chocolate Chip Almond Cookies 83

Chocolate Bark 84

No-Sugar Coconut Bark 85

Gelatin Hearts...85

Gluten-Free Vanilla Cake & Cupcakes 87

Coconut Whipped Cream Frosting 88

Chocolate Whipped Cream Frosting..88

Raw Dehydrated Macaroons 89

Cinnamon Almond Macaroons 89

Chocolate Chip Macaroons 90

Pineapple Coconut Macaroons 90

Fermented Foods

Non-Dairy Fermented Beverages 93

Young Coconut Kefir 94

Hibiscus and Rose Hip Soda 94

Non- Dairy Fermented Foods 95

Nut Yogurt 95

Nut Cream Cheese (Strained Yogurt) 96

Vegetable and Fruit Kebabs with Nut Yogurt Dipping Sauce 96

Apple Kraut 99

Dairy/Fermented Dairy 100

Fermented Dairy 103

Yogurt 103

Variation: Raw Milk Yogurt 104

Whey/Cream Cheese 104

Condiments and Sauces **110**

Honey-Mustard Dipping Sauce 106

BBQ Dipping Sauce 106

GFCF Ranch Dressing Dip 106

No-Mato (Tomato-Free) Sauce 107

Cranberry Apple Pear Sauce 108

Pear Sauce or Apple Sauce 108

White Bean Hummus 109

Allergen-Free & Non-Toxic Art Supplies and Bonuses **115**

Gluten-Free Playdough 111

Resources **117**

Cooking To Heal 117

What Parents Are Learning 117

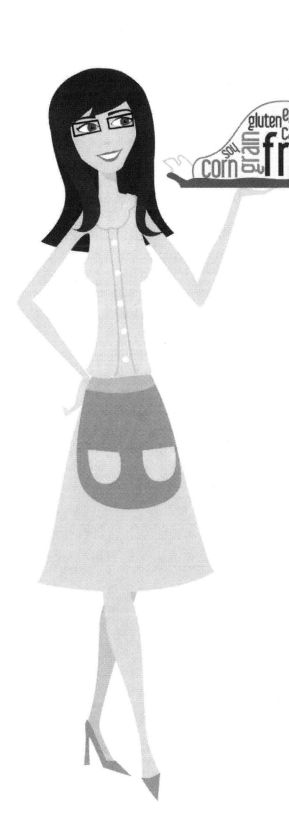

Nutrition and Diet

Diet Options
GFCF and SCD
Food Substances
Meal Planning
Tools of the Trade
Egg Substitutes

Why Special Diets?

Diet is a powerful tool. The choices we make about what to eat, and what to feed our children, have profound impact on health, and present great opportunity to support healing and recovery from autism.

Historically, autism was considered a "mysterious" brain disorder, implying that it begins and ends in the brain. Through the array of common physical symptoms observed and the breakthrough work of the Autism Research Institute, a more appropriate "whole body disorder" (the brain is affected by the biochemistry generated in the body) perspective of autism has emerged. Martha Herbert, M.D., Ph.D., who was one of the first to describe autism this way, refers to the brain as "downstream" from the body's functioning.

Common physical symptoms of children with autism include diarrhea, constipation, bloating and GI pain, frequent infections, sleeping challenges, and inflammation/pain. The systems often affected in autism include: digestion, immune function/inflammation, and detoxification.

These weaknesses in physiological functioning can be directly tied to biochemical processes that are affected by diet—i.e., the absence of requisite nutrients and/or the presence of offending substances. For many children, imbalances in these systems create nutrient deficiencies, food reaction, and underscores the importance of clean, organic, easy to digest food, free of food intolerances.

Altering food choices affects these processes and helps improve symptoms. This is why special healing diets are recommended and why cooking to heal is essential.

Nutrition and Diet

Digestion Connection

A healthy diet is essential for good health, and good digestion is critical.   Hippocrates, the father of modern medicine said, "All disease begins in the gut." A healthy GI tract provides the proper environment for good bacteria, proper enzyme function, and an ability to digest and absorb nutrients. We are not what we eat but what we can digest.

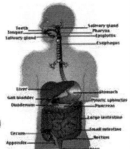

Many health conditions stem from, or are exacerbated by, impaired digestion and GI health. Poor digestion can lead to a condition known as leaky gut, malabsorption of nutrients, inflammatory responses to foods that are not broken down, and be a burden to the detoxification system (from substances that are created by imbalanced gut bugs and not readily eliminated). Poor digestion can stem from environmental factors (as well as genetic susceptibility), overuse of antibiotics, and lack of beneficial bacteria, inflammation, and immune system response to certain foods.

Benefiting from Dietary Intervention

The following seemingly diverse group of conditions has similar underlying causes (as in the below autism example) and dietary strategies:

- Autism
- ADHD

Nutrition and Diet

- Asthma
- Allergies
- Autoimmune conditions
- Digestive disorders
- Yeast/Candida
- Chemical sensitivities

What is a Healing Diet?

- Avoids problematic foods and ingredients
- Increases nourishing and healing foods

Following the principles of a healing diet helps restore balance to the following body systems—common underlying causes too many neurological and inflammatory conditions:

- * Immune function
- * Inflammation/pain
- * Digestion
- * Detoxification

Autism example:

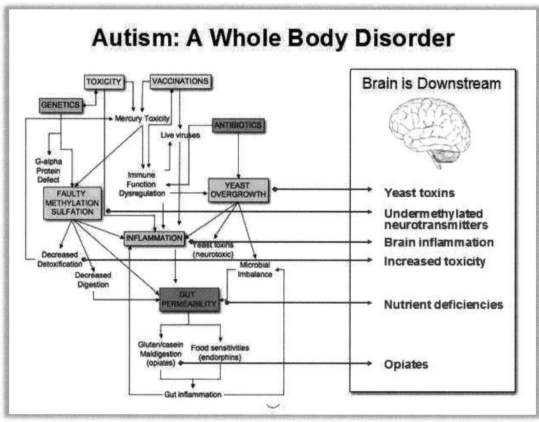

Taken from Nourishing Hope for Autism: Nutrition Intervention for Healing Our Children
Written by Julie Matthews, Certified Nutrition Consultant at NourishingHope.com

Nutrition and Diet

How Diet Can Help Support Digestion & Biochemistry

- Leaky Gut and Gut Inflammation
    - Remove foods that inflame gut
    - Add foods that heal gut
    - Add foods that supply beneficial bacteria
- Nutrient Deficiencies
    - Increase the quality of food and digestibility
- Yeast Overgrowth
    - Remove sugars
    - Remove starches
    - Add probiotic-rich foods
- Toxicity and Poor Detoxification
    - Avoid food additives
    - Avoid toxins in food supply and meal preparation
- Faulty Methylation and Sulfation
    - Remove phenolic foods
    - Improve methylation and sulfation through supplementation

People can reaction to many substances, additives, and ingredients in foods.

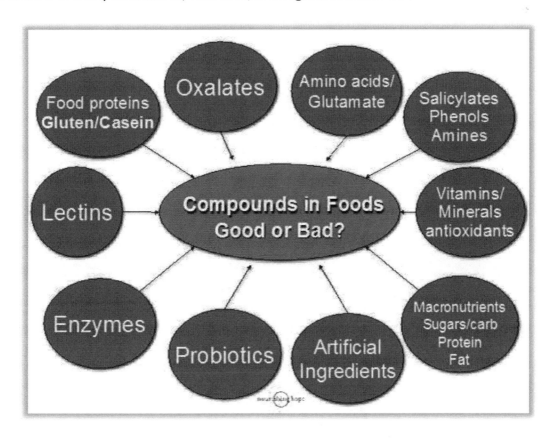

Nutrition and Diet

**Common food allergens/sensitivities can create inflammation and lead to digestion
And health problems:**

- Gluten: wheat, barley, rye, spelt, kamut, triticale, commercial oats
- Casein: all dairy products
- Soy
- Corn (even if you are not sensitive to corn, ONLY eat organic corn)
- Eggs
- Citrus
- Peanuts
- Chocolate
- Cane Sugar
- Beef

Diet Options	Benefits
GFCF (Gluten-free and Casein-free) No gluten (wheat, rye, barley, spelt, kamut, and commercial oats) or casein (dairy)	• Good diet to start with • Reduce gut inflammation • Reduce opiates
Food Sensitivity Elimination/Rotation Eliminating or rotating all other food sensitivities: Soy, corn, eggs, citrus, peanuts, chocolate, cane sugar, beef...	• Follow up on GFCF to refine food sensitivities
Feingold Diet/Low Phenols Restricts high phenolic foods, including all artificial ingredients and high salicylate fruits such as apples, red grapes, and berries	• Good diet for the following food addictions: grapes, apples, artificial ingredients • Common reactions: Hyperactivity, behavior, irritability, red cheeks
SCD (Specific Carbohydrate Diet)/GAPS Restricts carbohydrates to only fruits, non-starchy vegetables, and honey. No grains, starchy vegetables, or mucilaginous fiber	• Helpful for severe gut inflammation • Helpful for diarrhea/constipation not addressed by GFCF • Starves out dysbiotic flora
Body Ecology Diet™ Anti-yeast diet combining principles of anti-yeast diets including no sugar, acid/alkaline, fermented foods	• Great for ridding candida • Populating good bacteria
Low Oxalate Diet Restricts high oxalate foods (nuts, beans, greens)	• Helpful for pain-related conditions such as fibromyalgia. • Reduces inflammatory oxalates aiding gut healing and reduction of yeast/dysbiosis
Nourishing Traditions/ Weston A. Price Good quality fats, soaking and fermenting for digestion	• Nourishing diet • High quality fats, fermented foods, nutrient dense

Nutrition and Diet

Gluten-Free and Casein-Free (GFCF) Cooking

Sources of GLUTEN to avoid (unless specified gluten-free)	Sources of CASEIN to avoid
• Wheat	• All milk products (cow, goat, sheep)
• Rye	• Cheese
• Barley	• Yogurt
• Spelt	• Butter
• Kamut	• Buttermilk
• Triticale	• Ice cream
• Oats (commercial)	• Kefir
• Semolina	• Cream
• Hydrolyzed Vegetable Proteins	• Sour cream
• MSG	• Whey
• Dextrin	• Galactose
• Malt	• Casein, Caseinate
• Citric acid	• Lactose in seasoning
• Artificial flavors & coloring	• Lactalbumin as natural flavor
• "Spices"	• Lactic acid
• Soy sauce (unless wheat-free)	• Sherbet
• Potato chips/fries	• Canned tuna
• Sauces and gravies	• Cool Whip
• Bologna and hot dogs	• Artificial butter flavor
	• Milk chocolate
	• Wax on some fruits and vegetables
	• Seasoned potato chips
	• Hot dogs and bologna (may contain)

Substitutions for gluten	Substitutions for dairy
Rice	Milk & Yogurts
Millet	Rice milk
Quinoa	Almond, hazelnut or hemp milk
Amaranth	Homemade Nut milk
Buckwheat	Coconut milk
Corn	Potato milk
Wild rice	
Montina	Oil/Butter
Teff	Coconut oil
Sorghum	Ghee (certified casein-free brand)
Tapioca	Lard or tallow
Nut flours	Earth Balance

Nutrition and Diet

Seed flours	
Coconut flour	
Chestnut flour	Kosher items
Bean flours	Pareve only
Roots (taro, yam)	
Yucca/casava	Cheeses (soy-free brands)
• Non-gluten pasta (corn, rice, soba noodles (buckwheat))	Galaxy Foods' Rice Vegan Cheese Daiya Cheese
• Non-gluten bread (millet, rice bread)	
• Mochi (chewy rice baked item)	Ice Cream
Thickeners	Sorbets w/o milk
Agar	Non-dairy ice cream (rice or nut milk)
Guar gum	Coconut ice cream (Coconut Bliss)
Gelatin	Fruit popsicles
Kudzu powder	
Tapioca	Chocolate
Sweet rice flour	GFCF chocolate
Xanthan gum	
Arrowroot	

Spices, vinegar, and other ingredients may contain gluten so be sure to check your source.

Herbs and Spices
Good quality herbs and spice brands such as Frontier, Penzy, even McCormick are gluten-free for the most part. For these brands, herbs and spices that are single spices such as "basil," "cinnamon," or "onion powder," are gluten-free. However, spice *blends*, even for these higher end brands, are typically <u>not</u> gluten-free, such as apple pie spice, Mexican seasoning, and chili powder (which is a blend of chilies).

Vinegars
Malt vinegar is made from barley and is not gluten-free. Be careful of flavored vinegars, as these may contain gluten. Be careful at restaurants that might use cheap brands of vinegar that contain added colors or flavors that may contain gluten. Most vinegar in the US is not made from wheat, but from corn, apples, or some other substance. White vinegar or "vinegar" are typically distilled, and therefore gluten-free. Heinz white vinegar is gluten-free (and made from corn). Rice vinegar, apple cider vinegar, red and white wine vinegars, and balsamic vinegar are gluten-free.

Mustard is made with vinegar so you'll want to check with the brand to ensure its gluten-free. French's mustard is gluten-free. Dijon mustard is also gluten-free. However, always check with the company on mustard to confirm they don't use any gluten-containing ingredients.

Vanilla extract may or may not be gluten-free depending on the alcohol used. Frontier and McCormick's are gluten-free and most gluten-free vanilla says so right on the label.

GFCF Implementation Steps

Beginning GFCF

- Before removing anything, introduce GFCF alternatives such as rice pasta, GF waffles, and other GFCF foods and snacks. This will support the elimination portion later.
- Start eliminating **one at a time:**
  - Try casein-free for two to three weeks
  - Then remove gluten and continue both for three to six months
- Substitute same foods child likes with gluten/casein-free options. For example, if they eat waffles every morning, buy rice flour waffles.
- Do not increase the amount of sugar in the diet. It is common to start substituting *anything* gluten-free including high sugar cookies. If you need to continue to use some higher sugar foods (if they are already in the diet) during the transition, it is fine; however, you will want to take them out as soon as possible. Therefore, it's best to avoid them as much as possible, and avoid inadvertently introducing more.

GFCF Tips

- If the package does not say "gluten-free" and "casein-free," call manufacturer. Wheat-free and dairy-free, do not mean GFCF. Even if there are no gluten or casein ingredients, you can not assume GFCF due to trace ingredients and cross contamination that do not need to be listed.
- Try some prepared foods and mixes
- For younger kids, try putting gluten- and casein-free options in the old containers, i.e. put rice milk in the milk container.
- Add a digestive enzyme with DPPIV (see resource section). It is not a substitute for GFCF diet but will support it.

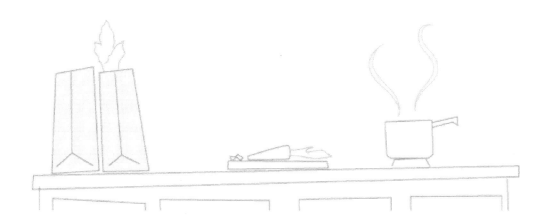

Nutrition and Diet

Specific Carbohydrate Diet (SCD) & Gut and Psychology Syndrome (GAPS) Diet

The GAPS diet is based on the Specific Carbohydrate Diet, so or the purpose of the cookbook, these diets will simply be tagged as "SCD" in the recipes.

While there are some differences in the diets, there are very few differences in the foods, with the exception that GAPS does not recommend baking soda while SCD allows it. Therefore, the baked goods "tagged" SCD that include baking soda, may not be appropriate for people on GAPS.

The following are some of the guidelines for SCD/GAPS. For more thorough examination, visit *Nourishing Hope for Autism*.

Foods to avoid on SCD/GAPS
- No grains, or foods make from grains such as pasta
- No rice or potato milk
- No corn
- No potatoes (white or sweet)
- No beans unless specified as allowable
- No soy products
- No cane sugar or molasses
- No corn syrup, high fructose corn syrup, or powdered fructose
- No maple syrup or agave nectar
- No artificial sweeteners (including sucralose or Splenda)
- No stevia
- No garlic and onion powder
- No cornstarch, arrowroot powder, tapioca, agar-agar or carrageenan
- No pectin in making jellies and jams
- No chocolate or carob
- No baking powder (baking soda is fine on SCD but not recommended on GAPS)
- Many supplements are not allowed because of SCD non-compliant fillers

Allowable SCD/GAPS foods (if no prior sensitivity)
- Non-starchy vegetables
- Fruit and 100% fruit juice not from concentrate
- Nuts
- Nut milk and coconut milk (homemade)
- Some beans: Dried white (navy) beans, lentils, split peas, lima beans
- Honey
- Meat and poultry

- Fish
- Eggs
- Coconut oil
- Oils made from grains such as corn oil and soybean oil are permitted (but not ideal)
- Ghee
- Lard
- Spices (of any kind except mixtures like apple pie spice and curry powder)
- Natural cheeses (if not casein intolerant)
- Homemade yogurt (if not casein intolerant)

Paleo

The Paleolithic or "Paleo" diet is what our ancestors the hunters and gatherers ate – the people and diet we evolved from. This diet consists of eating:
- Meats
- Organ meat
- Bone broth
- Eggs
- Vegetables
- Fruit
- Natural plant oils and animal fats
- Small amounts of starchy "tubers" or potatoes
- Small amounts of nuts and seeds

This diet does not include grains, beans, refined sugar or dairy. Paleo is another form of grain-free diet, different and distinct from SCD/GAPS. Paleo allows sweet potato but avoids beans, while SCD/GAPS allow certain beans while avoiding sweet potatoes.

Low Oxalate Diet (LOD)

The low oxalate diet (LOD) consists of low oxalate foods and keeping total oxalate under a certain amount. Officially, the diet counts milligrams of oxalates and keeps them between 40-60 mg for a 2000-calorie diet. That level is adjusted based on the calories in the diet, so that for a child with a lower calorie diet, the amount of oxalate is less. Some people choose to select mostly "low" oxalate foods with a few "medium" oxalates versus counting exact milligrams everyday. It's helpful to calculate the milligrams of oxalate for a day to two to ensure you are in the proper range, and then choose foods based on their general level. For more information on LOD see *Nourishing Hope for Autism*. For exact oxalate levels for foods see the Vulvar Pain Foundation's cookbook, the Trying_low_oxalates Yahoo Group, or other online resources listed in the back of the workbook. Recipes tagged LOD are not necessary all low oxalate ingredients, but they are "lower" oxalates foods (typically very low to medium) that can be part of a low oxalate diet (as long as total oxalate is keep within range).

Nutrition and Diet

Body Ecology Diet™ (BED)

The Body Ecology Diet (BED) incorporates many dietary principles. In addition to being low in sugars and only using certain grains (quinoa, millet, buckwheat and amaranth), it also involves the concepts of food combining, alkalizing, and fermented foods.

With food combining, BED pairs starches with vegetables, or meat with vegetables, but not meat and starches together. Generally, vegetables and other mineral-rich foods are alkalizing. There are more details on BED in *Nourishing Hope for Autism*. Recipes in this workbook contain alkalizing ingredients, fermented foods, and proper food combining. When building a meal, remember to properly combine foods. In other words, some BED recipes are meats and vegetables, others are starches and vegetables. To follow BED, remember not to include meat and starch recipes in the same meal. There are additional food combining principles—see http://www.bodyecology.com/07/01/18/food_combining_optimal_health_and_weight.php for more information.

Soaked almonds and seeds (except sesame) are allowed. Ocean vegetables (seaweeds), sour fruits (lemon, line, unsweetened cranberries and black currants) are allowed. Raw apple cider vinegar is used. Ghee is allowed and raw butter is often added.

Breads and flour products, yeast, sugars and mushrooms are not allowed on the diet. Beans and peanuts are not allowed on BED.

The principles of BED are complex. Refer to the Body Ecology book and website for details on how to follow this diet.

Feingold Diet (FG)

The **Feingold Diet** is the most basic diet that restricts salicylates and phenols. It avoids artificial ingredients such as: artificial colors, artificial flavors, the preservatives BHA, BHT, TBHQ, and aspartame and other artificial sweeteners.   It restricts many of the most commonly reactive salicylates such as almonds, apples, apricots, berries, cucumber, curry spices and most spices, grapes and raisins, oranges, honey, peaches, peppers, and tomatoes. Not every child will need to avoid all of the salicylates. This diet is customized to individual tolerances. See the complete list in the next section under "Feingold—High Salicylate Foods."

Failsafe Diet (FS)

The **Failsafe Diet** removes phenols and salicylates (more thoroughly than the Feingold Diet), as well as amines and glutamates, including MSG and food based forms (free glutamate). For a thorough list of high salicylate foods that are incorporated in the Failsafe diet there are several sources. *Nourishing Hope for Autism* has a chart in the appendix section on high salicylates according to research by Swain. Also Friendly Food by Swain, Soutter and Loblay has a great list of all of the Failsafe chemicals in foods. Failsafe also removes additional food additives including propionic acid, used in preserving bread and dairy products, and found by Derrick MacFabe, M.D. in rat studies to cause similar behavioral and biochemical symptoms that are found in autism (MacFabe 2007).

1212121212

Nutrition and Diet

Food Substances

Some food substances/chemicals that are artificial, and even natural, can cause problems for some individuals. Artificial ingredients are toxins and need to be detoxified—this adds burden to an often already overburdened system. Artificial additives are unhealthy for everyone and should be avoided. In the case of natural substances that occur in plants such as salicylates, amines, glutamates, and oxalates, certain people may be sensitive to them because of their biochemistry or unable to break them down. These foods are not by nature harmful, but can be problematic if someone cannot process them.

A few of the additives to always avoid and sources (there are often dozens or hundreds of sources, listed are some of the more common as examples):

- Avoid all MSG
    - Monosodium glutamate, Glutamate and Glutamic acid
    - Yeast nutrient, Yeast extract, Yeast food, and Autolyzed yeast
    - Hydrolyzed protein (any protein that is hydrolyzed) OR Hydrolyzed corn gluten
    - Gelatin
    - Calcium caseinate or Sodium caseinate
    - Textured protein
    - Monopotassium glutamate
- Trans-fats: partially hydrogenated fat,
- High fructose corn syrup
- Avoid all artificial colors (yellow #40, red#5, etc) and flavors
- Preservatives, flavorings, BHA, BHT, TBHQ, propionic acid (propionate)
- Nitrates/nitrites
- Sulfites
- Avoid artificial sweeteners: NutraSweet, Equal, aspartame, Sweet 'N Low, saccharine, sucrolose, Splenda.

Additives	Sources
MSG	Broths, soups, vegetarian meat products, gravy, cheese flavored crackers and chips
Trans-fats	Margarine, commercial peanut butter, commercial mayonnaise, fried foods, crackers and cookies
High fructose corn syrup	Jam, sodas, candy, cookies, almost anything sweetened could have it
Artificial colors and flavors	Candy, cereal, even possibly commercial yogurt
Preservatives	Bread, crackers, baked goods, milk
Nitrates/nitrites	Lunch meat, hotdogs, sausage
Sulfites	Dried fruit, dried apricots, prunes
Artificial sweeteners	Soda, gum, low calorie yogurt

Nutrition and Diet

In addition to the chemical additives, we all should avoid, the following are additional food chemicals (often naturally occurring) that many people want to avoid. Strong craving or addiction to any of the food substances below is a high indication that the food or group of substances is problematic.

Substance	Reaction	Who may benefit from removal
Phenols	Artificial colors and additives can trigger asthma, migraine headaches, and any of the salicylate reactions below.	ADHD, asthma, allergies, autism, and autoimmune conditions
Salicylates	Difficult to process if you have poor sulfation or methylation, such as in autism and lupus (research by Dr. Rosemary Waring). Hyperactivity, irritability, aggression, red cheeks/ears, sleep challenges	Many of those with autism, ADHD, asthma, as well as possibly lupus, rheumatoid arthritis, and other autoimmune may need to limit or avoid salicylates.
Amines/histamines	Migraine headaches trigger histamine/allergy response, sinus headache, irritability, sleep problems, heart palpitations.	Multiple chemical sensitivities, fibromyalgia, bipolar, and sensitive people such as those with autism may need to limit or avoid
Glutamates/MSG	Headaches, blurred vision, hyperactivity, diarrhea, panic attacks, anxiety, bags under eyes	Multiple chemical sensitivities, ADHD, asthma and sensitive people may need to avoid
Oxalates	Pain, urinary tract irritation, gut inflammation	Autoimmune conditions especially those with pain such as fibromyalgia, autism, interstitial cystitis, chronic pain conditions, vulvar pain, digestive disorders that are not improving, and an individual with a high oxalate diet and leaky gut

Nutrition and Diet

Chemical Phenols

- Artificial colors
- Artificial flavors: including Vanillin
- Preservatives – BHA, BHT, TBHQ

Feingold—High Salicylate Foods

- Almonds
- Apples
- Apricots
- Berries, raspberries, cherries
- Chili powder
- Cider and cider vinegar
- Cloves
- Coffee
- Cola drinks
- Cucumbers and pickles
- Curry powder
- Endive
- Grapes, raisins, currants

- Honey
- Nectarines and peaches
- Oranges and oranges
- Paprika
- Peppers (bell and chili)
- Pineapple
- Plums and prunes
- Radishes
- Tea
- Tomatoes
- Wine and wine vinegar
- Oil of wintergreen

Amines

Tyramine	Phenylethylamine	Histamine
- Aged or blue cheese - Yogurt - Smoked, cured or pickled meat or fish - Red wine or beer - Soy sauce, miso, tempeh	- Cheesecake - Yellow cheeses - Citrus fruit - Chocolate - Cocoa - Berry pie filling or canned berries - Red wine	- Banana - Beef, pork - Beer - Cheese, especially yellow ripened - Chicken liver - Eggplant - Fish, shellfish - Processed meat, such as salami - Sauerkraut - Tempeh, tofu, miso, tamari - Spinach - Strawberry - Tomato, tomato sauce, tomato paste - Wine - Yeast and foods containing yeast - Pineapple - Citrus fruit - Chocolate

Nutrition and Diet

Nightshades:

Be aware that nightshades can create inflammation and be a problem for some people. They are particularly associated with arthritis. While I'm not directly addressing nightshades in this book, you may want to remove them as well, especially if they are used frequently in the diet. Nightshades include: Tomatoes, eggplant, peppers (all types except peppercorns), and potatoes, as well as goji berries and gooseberries.

Glutamate	
MSG Additives	**Free Glutamate Naturally in food**
<ul><li>Monosodium glutamate, Glutamate and Glutamic acid</li><li>Yeast nutrient, Yeast extract, Yeast food, and Autolyzed yeast</li><li>Hydrolyzed protein (any protein that is hydrolyzed)</li><li>Hydrolyzed corn gluten</li><li>Gelatin</li><li>Calcium caseinate</li><li>Textured protein</li><li>Monopotassium glutamate</li><li>Sodium caseinate</li></ul>	<ul><li>Soy sauce</li><li>Roquefort cheese</li><li>Parmesan cheese</li><li>Grape juice</li><li>Tomatoes</li><li>Peas</li><li>Corn</li><li>Vegemite</li><li>Marmite</li><li>Gelatin/bone broth</li></ul>

High Oxalates Grains, beans, nuts, certain fruits and vegetables	
<ul><li>Beans (most – except black-eyed peas & yellow split peas are low. Garbanzo, lentils, Lima, and mung are medium.</li><li>Beets - tops, roots, greens</li><li>Berries (Blackberries, Raspberries)</li><li>Celery</li><li>Chocolate and Cocoa</li><li>Currants, red</li><li>Eggplant</li><li>Escarole</li><li>Figs, dried</li><li>Grains, especially buckwheat & millet (except white rice, wild rice, and corn)</li><li>Grapes, Concord</li></ul>	<ul><li>Nuts (all)</li><li>Okra</li><li>Parsley</li><li>Parsnips</li><li>Peppers, green</li><li>Pokeweed</li><li>Potatoes</li><li>Potatoes, sweet</li><li>Rhubarb</li><li>Rutabagas</li><li>Seeds (most – except pumpkin seeds, and sunflower seeds (medium))</li><li>Sorrel</li><li>Soybean</li></ul>

Nutrition and Diet

▪ Kiwi	▪ Spinach
▪ Leafy greens (Dandelion greens, Swiss chard, turnip greens, spinach) Collard, kale, and mustard greens are medium.	▪ Squash, yellow, summer
	▪ Tomato sauce, canned
	▪ Watercress
▪ Leeks	▪ Wheat, kamut, spelt
▪ Lemon, lime, orange peel	▪ Yams

Acceptable low oxalate "seeds" and flours (low and medium level): Pumpkin seeds, sunflower seeds, chestnuts, black-eyed peas, lentils, white rice, wild rice, coconut flour.

Meal Planning

Preparation Tips:

Breakfast
- Cook extra oatmeal. Next day, add a bit of water and as you heat it, the texture will return. You can do the same with bacon – just reheat.
- Cook extra vegetables to have some ready for vegetable omelet or scramble in AM, cooked sweet potatoes can be sliced and pan-fried.
- Make pancake blend of dry ingredients. Make up batch for a couple days and store batter in frig.
- Cook egg pie for several days.

Lunch
- Cook enough dinner for leftovers for lunch for self or kids.
- Cook extra meat you can use in something else the next day. For example, leftover drumsticks make a good snack; meatloaf can be used in a sandwich.

Dinner
- Cook enough grain (i.e. brown rice, quinoa) for a second meal.
- Chop vegetables for several days and put in containers in the refrigerator for quick addition for dinners, and as raw snacks.

General
- Cook a large soup, stew, chili, or casserole on Sunday or other free day. Freeze the leftovers for future dinners or lunches.
- Wash fruits so they are ready to grab and go
- Pre-grind flaxseeds or buy already milled flax seeds. Put in airtight container in freezer.
- Make a nut mixture (pre-grind nuts for smoothies, oatmeal, etc). Store in freezer.
- Make a GF flour blend.

Meal Planning Suggestions:
- Find a cooking buddy – someone you can commit to cooking with. If possible, find childcare. Make it fun—some clients even have a little wine while cooking and make it a social event. Cook large portions together and split dishes.

Nutrition and Diet

- Swap/share dishes. For example, one person can make a big batch of raw sauerkraut while the other makes a bone broth.
- Cook at least one large meal per week that you can eat two or three times as lunch or dinner.
- Make a meal plan. As simple as chicken on Monday and a beef dish on Tuesday, or make a more detailed plan with meals and even shopping lists. For rotation diets, you can create one or two weeks of rotation, and use a shopping list when you do your grocery shopping.
- Make a list of meal options to choose from (and have a line to add more) so you don't have to think of something new each day.

Meal Ideas

Breakfast

- Eggs, any style
- Breakfast meat with no nitrates/nitrites
- GFCF/SCD pancake, waffle, toast, or cereal (with a side of protein)
- French toast (GF bread)
- Fruit smoothie
    o Rice/nut milk, frozen fruit such as blueberries, pear, bananas, peaches, 1 tablespoon melted coconut oil, protein powder (rice or pea)

Lunch/Dinner

- Have a protein, vegetable, and starch, or "mock-starch" (the starch is not necessary and eliminated on certain diets such as SCD)
- Protein
    o Meatballs/meatloaf - Ground beef, buffalo, lamb or any meat
    o Burger – Ground chicken, beef, turkey, or other meat
    o Bean burger
    o Bean or lentil dish
    o Egg dish for dinner
    o GFCF, nitrate/nitrite-free hotdog and sausage
    o Homemade GF chicken nuggets
    o Any roasted chicken or meat
    o Chicken pancakes
    o Chicken sticks
- Vegetables
    o Steamed or boiled vegetables with ghee or coconut oil melted on top
    o Stir-fry vegetables
    o Salad
    o Raw sauerkraut
    o Crispy kale
- Starch

Nutrition and Diet

- o GF pasta – rice pasta, 100% buckwheat pasta, corn-quinoa pasta
- o Sweet potato or sweet potato fries or chips
- o Rice, quinoa, or millet dish
- o Dahl or bean dish
- Mock-starch (SCD-compliant)
  - o Cauliflower rice
  - o Cauliflower mashed "potatoes"
  - o Butternut squash fries
  - o Zucchini "noodles"
  - o Fruit (SCD carb)
- Additional lunch and dinner ideas
  - o Stews
  - o Casseroles
  - o Soup – Pureed or broth soup

Snacks

- Celery or apple with nut or seed butter
- Soaked almonds with fresh or dried fruit (no sulfites) with nuts
- Vegetables with hummus/SCD white bean hummus
- Chicken legs from dinner
- Smoothie (or frozen into popsicles)
- Vegetable juice (fresh made)
- French toast strips with coconut oil and a bit of salt (not sweet if possible)
- Chickpea snack
- Crispy kale
- Chicken or squash pancake

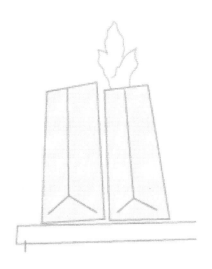

Tools of the Trade

Cooking

Cast iron and enameled cast iron are good options for cookware. Stainless steel pots and pans are also good options; however, stainless steel can contain high levels of nickel. Buy stainless steel that attracts a magnet—these are much lower in nickel. If you can find the old VisionWare by Corning Ware, they are also great to cook with. Do not use aluminum (where the cooking surface is aluminum), Teflon-coated, or copper. Especially, do not use Teflon. While they are easy and non-stick, there have been many studies showing this material is toxic. Even if they are new and unscratched, do not use them.

Toxins around the Kitchen	Safer Cooking Alternatives
Avoid aluminum cans	Buy in glass
Avoid storing in plastic	Store in glass w/metal or plastic lid
Avoid Teflon, copper, and aluminum pans	Use stainless steel (attracts a magnet), cast iron or enameled cast iron
Avoid the microwave, do not reheat in plastic	Heat in oven or on stove
Avoid plastic wrap & aluminum foil	Use wax paper or glass with lid

I highly recommend not using a microwave. Begin to heat food in a pot or pan on the stove, the oven, or a toaster oven. You will quickly begin to see that you really don't need and won't miss the microwave.

Store food in freezer-safe mason jars, glass or Pyrex storage containers. It is fine if the lid is plastic or rubber as it will typically not come in contact with the food. Wrap food in parchment paper before wrapping it in aluminum foil to avoid direct contact but to help hold shape.

Helpful Tools

Vitamix™: High powered blender that blends with ease. I suggest the grain attachment too. Grinding your own grain allows the flour to be very fresh.

Food Processor: Essential tool in my kitchen. A food processor is inexpensive and very versatile.

Excalibur™ Dehydrator: Great for making crispy nuts, dried fruit, SCD crackers, even yogurt (because you can adjust the temperature very specifically).

Harsch™ Crock: Unsurpassed for making lactic acid fermentations (cultured vegetables!). Healthy, easy to use. Makes great raw sauerkraut every time. Well worth the investment, but not necessary to make cultured vegetables.

Juicer: There are several different types of juicers: centrifugal and masticating being two of the most popular. See a comparison chart on juicers at: ttp://www.discountjuicers.com/compare.html

Thermos™: Great tool for hot lunches without having to use the microwave and when there is no way to heat up lunch when away from home.

Eggs and Egg Substitutes

Many people are sensitive or allergic to eggs. This can make cooking, especially baking, challenging.

Some people are intolerant to chicken eggs, but may tolerate duck or quail eggs. People sensitive to chicken eggs should be very cautious when trying duck or quail eggs. Do not try *any* eggs when there is a strong allergenic (IgE) response to chicken eggs—this could be dangerous with anaphylactic response. When using quail eggs, substitute them at a 5 to 1 ratio for large chicken eggs. Individuals with mild egg sensitivities may be able to rotate chicken eggs once every 3 or 4 days; others rotate duck, chicken, and quail eggs for reduced consumption of chicken eggs.

If eggs are not tolerated, try some of the following substitutions.

Eggs as Leavening Agents

The following helps with recipes for foods such as pancakes or cakes that need to rise.

Egg Replacer by Ener-G Foods
GFCF
Contains processed ingredients and not allowed on certain diets - not SCD compliant.
1 1/2 Tablespoons Egg replacer + 2 tablespoons water mixed well = 1 egg

No Egg by Orgran
GFCF

Similar to Egg Replacer

Baking Soda and Water
GFCF/ SCD/GAPS/Paleo/LOD/BED

Good for most diets. However, it's a bit tricky and doesn't work with all recipes, especially where a large number of eggs are needed.

1 1/2 TBL water
1 1/2 TBL oil
1 tsp baking soda
1/2 tsp vinegar (optional)
= 1 egg

Whisk above ingredients together in a cup and pour into mixture that calls for an egg. Adding the vinegar should provide a bit more rising power but is not necessary and may add strange flavor depending on the dish. This will not work for replacing a large number of eggs (more than 3) because the baking soda will make the recipe too bitter.

Acidic agents such as lemon juice and vinegar help boost the leavening process. Baking powder and extra oil can also function as a leavener.

1 heaping tablespoon baking powder, 1 1/2 tablespoon water, plus 1 1/2 tablespoons oil.
Where corn-free baking powder is needed, use Featherweight Baking Powder.

Eggs as Binding Agents

Helps with recipes that need eggs to help ingredients stick together, as in a muffin, meatball, etc.

Flax Seed and Water (Flax Seeds Are Not SCD Compliant)
GFCF/GAPS/Paleo/LOD/BED

1 Tablespoon flax seed with 3 Tablespoons water. Blend in blender. = 1 egg
Chia seeds can be used in the same way.

Pureed Fruit or Vegetable
GFCF/ SCD/GAPS/Paleo/LOD/BED

Cooked and pureed squash or banana, or many other vegetables like cauliflower,
¼ cup = 1 egg

Gelatin
GFCF/ SCD/GAPS/PaleoLOD/BED

Mix one envelope of unflavored gelatin with 1 cup boiling water . One envelope should be ¼ ounce; you can also use 2 teaspoons of Bernard Jensen's gelatin (Radiant Life Catalog)

3 tablespoons of liquid replaces one egg. (Refrigerate leftover portion. Then, melt to liquefy before using)

Arrowroot Powder
GFCF

Can also be used as a binding agent. 2 Tablespoons arrowroot with a bit of liquid added to a recipe = 1 egg

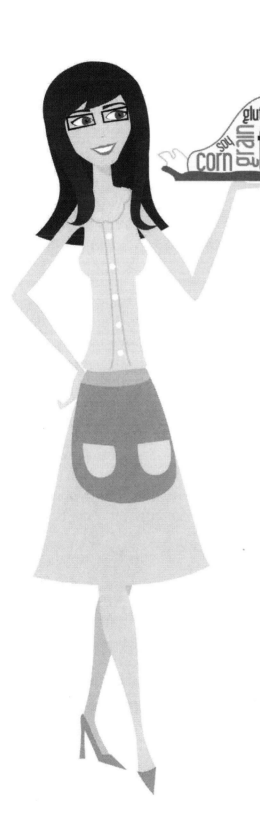

Nutrient Density

Vegetables
Stocks
Sneaking in Nutrients

Stocks/Soup Recipes
Vegetable Recipes
Juicing

Nutrient Density

Stocks and Broths

Consuming a nutrient dense diet is important for good health. It is particularly important with digestion and absorption problems where every nutrient counts. Stocks and broths are a simple way to boost nutrients in the diet.

Mineral-rich Stocks and Broths

Bone stocks and vegetable broths are great ways to increase consumption of highly absorbable nutrients. Using root vegetables, potato skins, carrots, celery, parsley, and seaweed, you can make a very nutrient-dense vegetable broth (or add these vegetables to a bone stock) that you can use to prepare soup, to cook rice, or even drink as a tea.

Bones stocks/broths are traditionally used by most native cultures as a way to nourish the sick, elderly, and mothers after childbirth. Grandma's old remedy of chicken soup when you're sick was based on a great deal of truth. The bones (of chicken, beef, lamb and other meats) add calcium, magnesium and potassium into the broth. The natural gelatin is wonderfully rejuvenating for digestion. The gelatin contains high levels of arginine and glycine (two important amino acids), and according to Sally Fallon, "acts as a 'protein sparer,' allowing the body to more fully utilize the complete proteins that are taken in" from other sources. This is important and advantageous for children who do not eat much protein. The addition of vegetables to these stocks adds electrolytes.

Minerals are absorbed in ionic form. If they are not in ionic form when consumed, they are ionized in the gut as salts dissolving into their two components or chelates releasing their key elements. Mineral-rich bone broths have all of the macro minerals--sodium, chloride, calcium, magnesium, phosphorus, potassium and sulfur available in ready-to-use ionized form as a true electrolyte solution.

Salt

When choosing salt, use an unrefined salt, such as Celtic brand sea salt or crystal salt (such as the Original Himalayan crystal salt). Unrefined salt is minimally processed, has dozens of trace minerals, and does not contain the additives and anti-caking agents that refined salt often has. Additionally, when unrefined salt is added to water or broth it supplies these minerals in ionic form (for easy absorption).

Always remember to get additional iodine from food or supplementation. While unrefined salt has some iodine, it may not be enough to meet nutritional needs alone. Kelp and multivitamin/mineral formulas are sources of iodine.

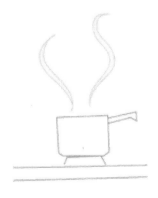

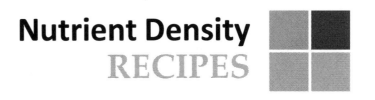

Nutrient Density RECIPES

Chicken Stock
GFCF/ SCD/GAPS/Paleo/LOD/BED/FG, Egg-Free/Nut-Free

To make LOD or to simplify, eliminate vegetables and make a simple bone broth, or use LOD vegetables.

Ingredients
1 whole pastured chicken
Gizzards, head and feet from one chicken (optional)
4 quarts cold filtered water
2 tablespoons vinegar
Add any vegetables desired

Directions
Cut whole chicken. Place into a large stainless steel pot with water and vinegar. Let stand 30 minutes to 45 minutes.

Add vegetables. Gently bring to a boil. Skim any scum that rises to the top. Reduce heat, cover and simmer for 6 to 24 hours.

1 ½ - 2 hours in, remove chicken that easily falls off the bone and use in chicken soup or a chicken dish. Add the greens 30 minutes before the stock is complete.

Strain the stock and cool in your refrigerator. Once fat has hardened and congeals on the top, scoop it off and save it for cooking. Store broth in refrigerator or freezer depending on length of storage.

Veggie Stock
GFCF/ SCD/GAPS/Paleo/LOD/BED/FG/FS, Egg-Free/Nut-Free

Can be made FG and FS with diet-compliant vegetables. Avoid the potatoes, sweet potatoes, and seaweed on SCD/GAPS and the potato on Paleo.

Try:
- Carrots
- The skins of potatoes
- Sweet potato
- Kale
- Parsley
- Nettles (be careful—fresh nettles sting until boiled, dried do not)
- Seaweed (kombu, wakame, dulse, etc)

Simmer chopped vegetables in a pot for 30-45 minutes. Strain vegetables and discard.

This recipe can be made GFCF, SCD/Gaps, BED or LOD depending on the vegetables used. Seaweed is not SCD/Gaps compliant.

Acorn or Butternut Squash Soup
GFCF/ SCD/GAPS/Paleo/BED/LOD/FG, Egg-Free/Nut-Free

For LOD, note that ginger is a little higher in oxalate than garlic.

To save time, use squash baked from the previous night's dinner.

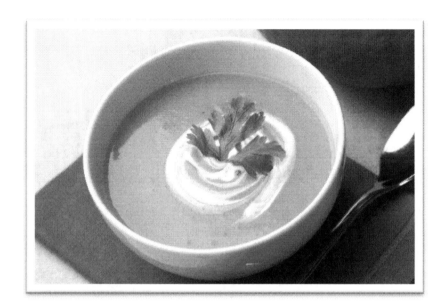

Ingredients
2 cups acorn or butternut squash
1 ½ cups chicken broth
½ cup onions
1 teaspoon minced garlic or ginger
1 teaspoon salt
Ghee or oil

Directions
Bake squash in oven: Cut squash in half length-wise and scoop out seeds. Place flat side down on baking dish with ½ inch of water on bottom and bake for 20-40 minutes until soft at 375 degrees. Pierce squash with fork prior to baking.

Sauté onions in ghee or other oil until soft, approximately 10-15 minutes. Add ginger or garlic in last few minutes of sautéing.

Add squash, broth, and salt. Puree with hand blender in pot or transfer to blender to blend. Heat the soup in pot until simmering.

Dress with a swirl of coconut cream and parsley leaf, if desired. Serve.

Stew
GFCF, Egg-Free/Nut-Free

Ingredients
Pastured beef (stew meat cuts) or lamb shank
1 pint of beef (or chicken) stock
8 oz of water
6 potatoes (chopped)
4 carrots (chopped)
2-3 parsnips (chopped)
1 head of cauliflower (chopped)
2 stalks celery (finely chopped)

1 small onion (finely chopped)
½ to 1 bunch of greens such as kale (finely chopped)

Directions
Place all ingredients (except greens) in a crock pot/slow cooker and cook for 6-8 hours – start on high until simmering (could take 5 or more hours), then turn down to low. In the last 30 minutes of cooking, add chopped greens/kale.

SCD Stew
GFCF/ SCD/GAPS/Paleo/BED/FG, Egg-Free/Nut-Free

Ingredients
Pastured beef (stew meat cuts) or lamb shank
1 pint of beef (or chicken) stock
8 oz of water
4 carrots
2 stalks of celery
2 heads of cauliflower
1 celery root
2 stalks celery (finely chopped)
1 small onion (finely chopped)
½ to 1 bunch of greens such as kale (finely chopped)

Directions
Place all ingredients (except greens) in a crock pot/slow cooker and cook for 6-8 hours – start on high until simmering (could take 5 or more hours), then turn down to low. In the last 30 minutes of cooking, add chopped greens/kale.

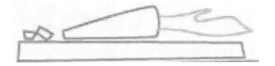

Kid-Friendly Vegetables
Sneaking Nutrients in the Diet

Everyone benefits from getting more nutrients in the diet. For kids that don't eat many vegetables, sneaking nutrients into meals can be a simple way to boost nutrient content in the diet.

Nutrient Boosting Strategies

- Use stock or broth as base for soup.
- Add a small dash of nutritive salt such as Celtic sea salt or Himalayan crystal salt to taste, especially in a broth.
- Add kombu, nettles or other green to cooking liquid of grains, beans, soups, or pasta.
- Simply soaking grains to increase digestibility will get more nutrients in the diet.
- Cook grains or pasta in chicken stock and vegetable broth.
- Add pureed meat and vegetables into various foods (as shown below).
- Sneak finely chopped vegetables to meatballs and various dishes (as shown below).
- Be creative with texture to help make vegetables appealing.

Stages of Sneaking

Stage One for Pickier Eaters
Puree very smooth and only start with a small amount, such as a tablespoon. Ease cautious eaters into it by using a small amount so they won't really notice it. Use these foods in anything—pancakes, muffins, smoothies, meat, sauce. They are undetectable for the most part—nothing green at least.

Butternut or acorn squash
Carrots
Turnips
Cauliflower
Summer squash or zucchini (peeled)
Chicken

Stage Two Purees
These green and dark vegetables will be noticeable in some dishes. However, you can still disguise them such as beets in chocolate cake, and greens in meat or sauce.

Broccoli   Green beans
Beets   Kale
Peas

Stage Three – shredded or chopped
Vegetables prepared this way often work well in muffins, latkes, and meatloaf
Carrots – shredded

Nutrient Density
RECIPES

Beets – shredded
Broccoli – finely chopped
Zucchini – shredded
Kale – finely chopped
Onion – finely chopped

Work your way up in color, flavor, texture, and amount over time.   Try the following ingredients in these dishes...

Pancakes:
- Chicken
- Butternut/winter squash
- Sweet potato
- Cauliflower

Meatballs/loaf/burgers:
- Liver—pureed
- Greens—finely chopped
- Butternut/winter squash
- Carrots shredded or pureed
- Broccoli—finely chopped

Chicken "sticks": cauliflower

Bean burgers:
- Kale—finely chopped
- Carrots—chopped
- Onions—chopped

Smoothies:
- Vegetable juices
- Pureed vegetables such as:
  - butternut
  - carrots
  - turnips
  - cauliflower

Treats:
- Shredded beets in chocolate cake
- Pureed greens in chocolate cake
- Avocado as based for dairy-free pudding (see recipe in Desserts section

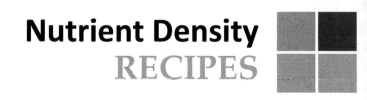

Making Purees

Cook food by steaming or roasting (such as butternut squash). Blend in blender or food processor until smooth with as little water as necessary (start with 1 tablespoon). Freeze in individual serving sizes such as half pints or ice cube trays.

Mashed Cauliflower "Potatoes"

GFCF/ SCD/GAPS/ Paleo/LOD/FG, Egg-Free/Nut-Free

This recipe is SCD/Gaps compliant. For those on GFCF and not SCD, you can use half potatoes—this way you have mashed potatoes with hidden cauliflower. For LOD, use coconut or rice milk. To make nut-free, use any nut/seed-free milk.

Ingredients
1 head cauliflower, or 1 pound frozen cauliflower florets
1/8-1/4 cup nut milk (or other CF milk)
1 tablespoon ghee
½ teaspoon salt

Directions
Boil or steam cauliflower until fork tender (10-20 minutes). Drain thoroughly (squeeze out excess water with a clean kitchen towel). Place cauliflower, milk, ghee and salt in food processor, blend until smooth.

You can bake mashed cauliflower potatoes, if desired for an even better, and drier texture. Place blended cauliflower mixture into a baking dish. Bake at 350 degrees until dish is bubbling hot.

Variation: You can also make recipe with half potatoes to sneak in cauliflower for picky eaters. Cook potatoes along with cauliflower and follow recipe. You may work your way to 100% cauliflower or keep it 50/50.

Cauliflower Rice

GFCF/ SCD/GAPS/ Paleo/LOD/BED/FG, Egg-Free/Nut-Free

Ingredients

1 head cauliflower
1 tablespoon oil (olive oil works well)
Salt and freshly ground pepper (white pepper for LOD)

Directions
Pulse cauliflower in food processor until the size of rice—a few short pulses. Don't over blend into puree. Heat pan, add oil, then add cauliflower. Sauté for only a few minutes (3-5 minutes).

Nutrient Density
RECIPES

Roasted Cauliflower
GFCF/SCD/GAPS/Paleo/LOD/BED/FG, Egg-Free/Nut-Free

While roasting typically involves the oven, it's the process of getting it brown and caramelized that I'm referring to in the name. You can either "roast" the cauliflower in the oven or on the stove. I prefer the stove so I can watch it more closely.

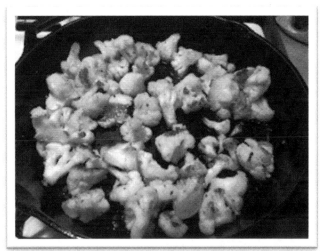

Ingredients
1 head of cauliflower
Coconut oil, refined (flavorless)
Unrefined salt

Directions
Wash cauliflower and break into pieces. I like some small crunchy bits so I break mine up into various sized small chunks.

Heat iron skillet or pan to medium-high. Add coconut oil, and then add cauliflower chunks. Sprinkle with salt. Stir occasionally so cauliflower has a chance to get browned, but not burnt. Cook cauliflower in pan for about 25 minutes, or until done.

Kale Chips
GFCF/ SCD/GAPS/ Paleo/LOD/BED/FG, Egg-Free/Nut-Free

You can also use other greens such as arugula (rocket), dandelion greens, mustard greens or others. Use lacinato kale for lower oxalate. Depending on the serving size, these kale chips are a low/medium oxalate food, that have a place in most low oxalate diets.

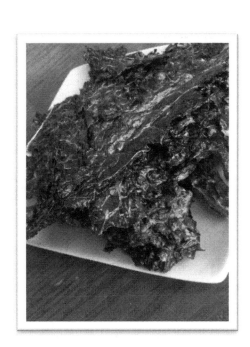

Ingredients
Bunch of Kale
Olive oil
Unrefined salt
Herbs and spices as desired (smoked paprika/capsicum, cayenne, rosemary or any)

Directions
Rinse kale leaves and dry. Remove stem of kale. Rub with olive oil. Season with salt and any other herbs you'd like.

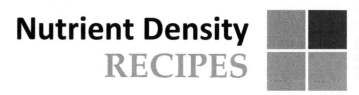
Heat oven to 325 degrees. Place stalks directly on oven rack and cook for 10-15 minutes. Watch closely so they don't burn. Chips should be green and crispy, not browned – browned is burnt.

Brussels Sprouts Chips
GFCF/ SCD/GAPS/ Paleo/LOD/BED/FG, Egg-Free/Nut-Free

Ingredients
Brussels Sprouts
Olive oil
Unrefined Salt (like Celtic brand Sea Salt or Himalayan Crystal salt)

Directions
Preheat oven to 350 degrees.

Wash Brussels sprouts, cut off end, and pull off larger leaves that you want to make chips with. Rub leaves with olive oil, place on baking sheet, and sprinkle with salt (and any other herbs you want). Place chips in oven to bake for 12-19 minutes. Depends on the oven and temperature. It's better to go lower and slower. If leaves are brown, they taste burnt—you want them mostly green. Between 325-350 degrees is good.

Zucchini Chips
GFCF/ SCD/GAPS/ Paleo/LOD/BED/FG, Egg-Free/Nut-Free

Ingredients
2-3 Zucchini (or summer squash)
Olive oil
Unrefined Salt (like Celtic brand Sea Salt or Himalayan Crystal salt)
Parchment paper

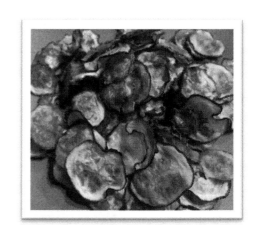

Directions
Preheat oven to 350 degrees.

Wash zucchini, cut off ends, and peel if desired. Thinly slice with mandolin if you have one, or a knife or with a vegetable peeler. Slice into thin chips, and rub them with olive oil. Place on baking sheet with parchment paper (you need parchment or they will stick), and sprinkle with salt (and any other herbs you want).

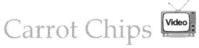

Carrot Chips

GFCF/ SCD/GAPS/ Paleo/BED/FG/FS, Egg-Free/Nut-Free

Ingredients
Carrots
Oil (Expeller-pressed coconut oil (Wilderness Family Naturals) or grass-fed lard)
Salt

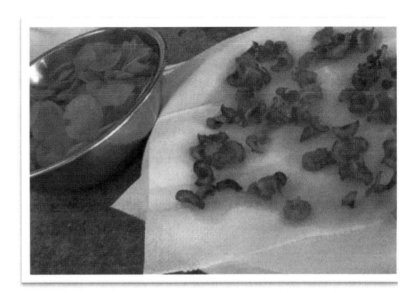

Directions
Cut carrots into thin discs or curls with a vegetable peeler. Deep fry in until lightly brown around edge. Remove from oil and place on paper towel to absorb excess oil. Salt chips.

They are still a little soggy when they first come out, but they will firm up as they cool.

You can use butternut squash, parsnips, or beets, as well as other vegetables (if dietary compliant). Parsnips are not SCD/Gaps.

Carrot Fries

GFCF/ SCD/GAPS/ Paleo/LOD

An iron skillet works great for this if you have one – the heat distributes and browns the carrots well without burning. Great for any root vegetables: carrot, parsnip, rutabaga/swede, etc. For low oxalate, choose low/medium oxalate root vegetables and portion sizes according to low oxalate needs (carrots are higher than parsnip or rutabaga/swede).

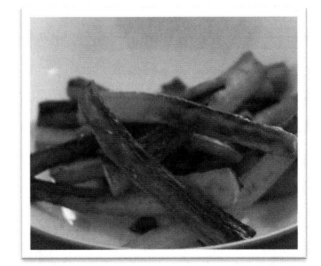

Ingredients
4 carrots (tender rainbow carrots are lovely for this)
Ghee (or expeller-pressed coconut oil)

Directions
Cut carrots in half length-wise. Then cut into thin wedges.

Heat iron skillet to medium-high and add ghee (or coconut oil). Add carrots. Brown on one side by leaving them for 5-10 minutes, then flip carrots and brown the other side. Be careful not to burn.

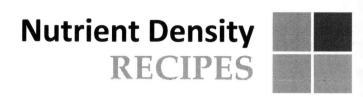

Winter Squash French Fries
GFCF/ SCD/GAPS/ Paleo/LOD/BED/FG/FS, Egg-Free/Nut-Free

Use acorn or butternut squash for LOD.

Ingredients
Butternut squash or other winter squash
Olive oil

Directions
Preheat oven to 425F. Cut butternut squash into thin slices by hand or with a slicer. Toss them in olive oil, and place slices on a *baking stone. Bake until crisp. No turning is required
Tip: Baking stone is available from Pampered Chef™

Butternut Hash Browns
GFCF/ SCD/GAPS/ Paleo/LOD/BED/FG/FS, Egg-Free/Nut-Free

Ingredients
Butternut Squash
Expeller-Pressed (Unflavored) coconut oil
Salt and pepper

Directions
Peel a butternut squash. Grate with a cheese grater.

Heat iron skillet or pan, add oil, and place haystacks of butternut squash into the pan.

Pan-fry on medium heat until browned and crispy. Flip. Sprinkle salt and pepper to taste.

Squash Pancakes
GFCF/ SCD/GAPS/ Paleo/LOD/BED/FG/FS
Nut-Free

Ingredients
1 cup pureed squash (acorn/butternut for LOD)
4 eggs
1 TBL melted coconut oil or ghee

Directions
Mix squash and eggs in food processor. Heat pan, add oil, and prepare as pancakes.

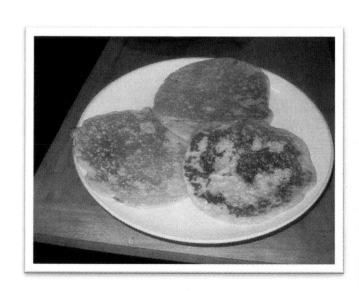

Nutrient Density
RECIPES

Banana Pancakes
GFCF/SCD/GAPS/Paleo/LOD/FG, Nut-free

Ingredients
3 ripe bananas with brown spots
2 pastured eggs
½ teaspoon vanilla extract
pinch (1/8 teaspoon) salt
Oil – Expeller-Pressed Coconut oil

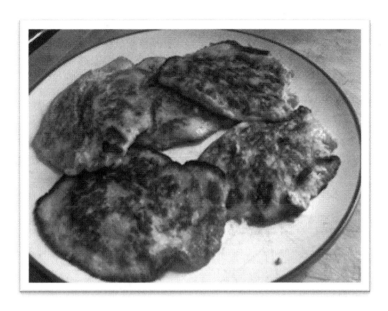

Mash bananas with fork. Beat in eggs. Add vanilla and salt and mix. Coat pan with oil. Spoon batter into pan. Cook on low so pancakes set before flipping to make turning pancakes easier. Cook until done.

Makes 8-10 pancakes.

Confetti Brussels Sprouts
GFCF/ SCD/GAPS/ Paleo/LOD/BED/FG/FS, Egg-Free/Nut-Free

FS without nuts or onion, and use ghee or sunflower oil.

To make LOD and nut-free, avoid pecans and other nuts. There is some controversy on oxalate level for Brussels sprouts depending on how they are cooked. Cut in half and boil Brussels sprouts for 5 minutes for LOD. This is a medium oxalate recipe. Use soaked almonds for BED.

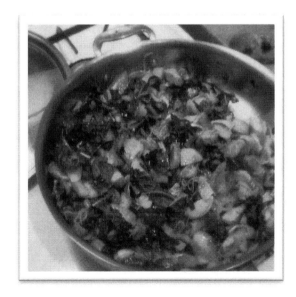

Ingredients
1 – 1½ lb Brussels sprouts
½ onion
½ cup pecans or other nuts
Refined (flavorless) coconut oil or ghee
Salt

Directions
Wash Brussels sprouts and cut off bottom and peel off a leaf or two if needed.   Put sprouts in food processor and pulse briefly into a confetti texture, do not over mince. Dump out finished sprouts and hand chop or pulse any remaining large pieces.

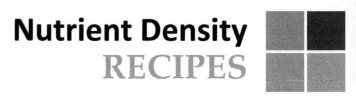

Dice onions and sauté in oil for 2-5 minutes and *begin* to caramelize onions. Add salt. Before onions are caramelized, add chopped Brussels sprouts and nuts to onions. Cook for 5 minutes or until Brussels sprouts and onions are ready.

Variation: Add dried cranberries or other dried fruit for a holiday dish. Dried cranberries would not be SCD/Gaps compliant.

Green Beans and Almonds
GFCF/ SCD/GAPS/ Paleo/BED/FG/FS, Egg-Free/Nut-Free

This recipe is similar to the Brussels sprouts recipe. FG/FS without nuts, and avoid onion on FS.

To make LOD, avoid almonds (Use sunflower or pumpkin seeds). To make nut free, eliminate the almonds.

Ingredients
1½ lb green (string) beans
½ onion, diced
½ cup chopped or slivered almonds
Ghee
Salt

Procedure
Dice onions and sauté with ghee for 2-5 minutes and *begin* to caramelize onions. Before onions are caramelized, add green beans, nuts, and salt (to taste). Cook for 10-20 minutes or until ready (some beans are tougher than others). Don't overcook.

Broccoli with Lemon and Sesame Seeds
GFCF/ SCD/GAPS/ Paleo/BED/FG, Egg-Free/Nut-Free

Skip the sesame seeds for BED.

Ingredients
1 bunch of broccoli
1/3 cup chopped shallot or onion
1/3 cup sesame seeds
Juice from ½ lemon
Salt

Directions
Toast sesame seeds in dry pan.   Set aside.

Sauté shallots or onions. Add broccoli and cook covered for 5 minutes. Uncover and cook for 15 minutes or until done. Squeeze on lemon juice (it should add "pizzazz" more than sour flavor). Add salt to taste. Sprinkle on toasted sesame seeds.

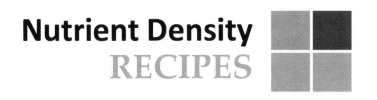

Vegetable Latkes
GFCF/ SCD/GAPS/ Paleo/LOD/BED/FG, Nut-Free

Ingredients
3 cups shredded zucchini
1 cauliflower
1 onion
2 eggs
salt/pepper (white pepper for LOD)
oil for pan-frying (Coconut or ghee)

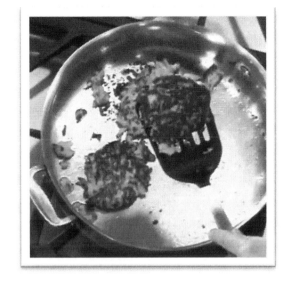

Directions
Place zucchini in a towel and twist out water. This is a crucial step. Let zucchini drain as much as possible. Cut cauliflower and steam until vegetable is soft – able to easily mash with a fork. If watery, place in towel and wring out water.

Heat oil and sauté onions until caramelized. For ease, skip the sautéing and use *raw* finely chopped onions.
Combine zucchini, cauliflower, and onions in bowl. Add eggs, salt and pepper. Mix with hands.

Heat until browned and egg is thoroughly cooked. Variation: Add other shredded vegetables such as carrots.

Potato and Vegetable Latkes
GFCF/FG, Nut-Free

Flour can be eliminated.

Ingredients
2 cups of shredded potatoes (potatoes can be peeled or with peel)
1 cup shredded vegetable (any, sweet potato, carrot, and zucchini)
1 onion, finely chopped
2 eggs
2 T. rice flour
1/2 teaspoon salt

Directions
Pat excess liquid from potatoes. Mix all ingredients in a bowl.
Heat pan, add oil such as ghee or lard to pan, Fry the pancakes until browned on each side. Best served hot.
Top with applesauce (avoid on Feingold diet) or pear sauce, if desired.
Variation: These potato latkes can also be made with 100% sweet potato instead of white potato.

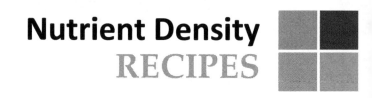

Beet Herb Salad with Pomegranate
GFCF/SCD/GAPS/Paleo, Nut-Free, Egg-Free

For SCD/GAPS and Paleo use honey in place of molasses.

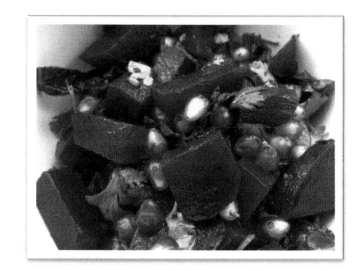

Ingredients
3-4 medium beets - one bunch
Seeds from one pomegranate
1/2 cup fresh cilantro leaves
1/4 cup chopped herbs such as mint, or kale leaves (I like to do fine strips of kale)
Juice from one lemon juice
1 tablespoons molasses
1/4 cup olive oil
1 teaspoon crushed red pepper flakes
½ teaspoon sea salt

Directions
Peel and chop beets. Boil beets for 40 minutes. Place in a medium bowl and cool down beets.
Pour the lemon juice and molasses into a bowl, whisk in the olive oil. Add the red pepper and salt and mix. Let is for 5 minutes.

Combine the beets, pomegranate seeds, cilantro, herbs and other greens, and toss with dressing.

Kale Salad
GFCF/SCD/GAPS/Paleo/LOD, Nut-Free, Egg-Free

For LOD use lacinato kale, and consider portion size to not overdue oxalates.

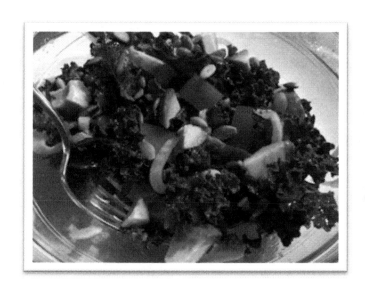

Ingredients
1 bunch kale –la cinato /dinosaur, curly green or red Russian kale
1 lemon, juiced
1/4 teaspoon salt
3 Tablespoons extra virgin olive oil
Shaved fennel
½ red pepper, chopped

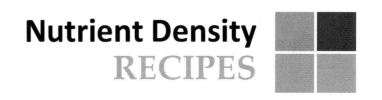
1 avocado, cut into pieces or slices
1/4 cup pumpkin seeds (raw or toasted)

Directions
Remove the kale stems from the leaves and chop them into small/medium-sized pieces. Pour a small bit of oil and lemon juice in a small bowl and put aside.

Massage in the lemon juice and salt with your hands. After a few minutes the leaves will become wilted, then rub on olive oil.

Shave fennel on mandolin or slice very thin. Add the fennel, red pepper, avocado, and mix.

Sprinkle pumpkin seeds on top, either raw or toasted. Wisk remaining oil and lemon juice, and drizzle over salad.

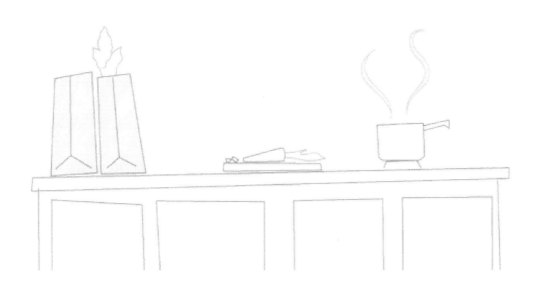

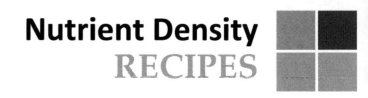

Juicing

Juicing is a wonderful way to add nutrients, chlorophyll, and enzymes to the body. Chlorophyll has a structure similar to hemoglobin, the substance in blood responsible for transporting oxygen. Juicing allows for a greater extraction and concentration of nutrients.

Base Vegetables

Use vegetables with a neutral flavor that can balance stronger flavored ones like broccoli, which may be difficult to drink straight up. Carrot is often used as a base, just be aware of its higher sugar content.

- Celery
- Cucumber
- Fennel
- Carrot

Healthy Accents

- Ginger
- Lemon
- Green apple
- Sour fruits
- Broccoli
- Kale
- Cabbage
- Collard greens

Sweet Fruits

Use sweet fruits and vegetables with strong vegetables like broccoli and kale to balance flavor.
- Apple
- Pear
- Melon
- Beet
- Carrot
- Berries

Add water to any juice that is too strong. Add natural sparkling water for a "soda" kids love.

All juicing recipes are Egg-Free/Nut-Free.

Cooking to Heal

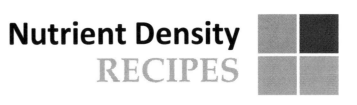

The Beginner Juice
GFCF/ SCD/Gaps/Paleo

2 carrots
1 apple
½ beet

Enzymes Juice
GFCF/ SCD/Gaps/Paleo

½ mango
1 cup papaya
1/8 chunk of large pineapple with rind
2 kiwis with skins

Digestion Juice
GFCF/ SCD/GAPS/BED/Paleo

½ inch piece ginger
5-10 sprigs of mint
2 kiwis with skins
½ fennel bulb

Potassium
GFCF/Paleo

5-10 sprigs parsley
1/4 jicama
Carrots
Spinach
Celery

Iron
GFCF/ SCD/Gaps/Paleo

2 leaves kale
½ cup broccoli
½ beet
2 carrots
1 orange

Anti-Inflammatory
GFCF/ SCD/GAPS/BED/Paleo

Use green apple instead of pineapple for BED.

¼ pineapple with rind
¼ inch piece of ginger
2 collard green leaves
½ fennel bulb
¼ inch piece of fresh turmeric root - optional

Antioxidants
GFCF/ SCD/Gaps/Paleo

1 apple
¼ cup blueberries
2 kiwis with skin
1 carrot
¼-½ red pepper

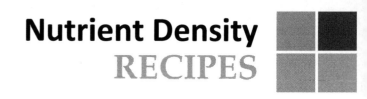

Smoothies

Green Smoothie
GFCF/SCD/GAPS/Paleo/LOD

Because of kale and these other low and medium oxalate ingredients, you can enjoy this green smoothie as part of a low oxalate diet. Choose low oxalate berries like strawberries and blueberries, and make sure to consider serving size to keep with a low oxalate diet.

Ingredients
1 cup mango (fresh or frozen)
1/2 cup berries (fresh or frozen)
1 banana
1/2 avocado
5 kale leaves de-stemmed (about one cup of kale)
12 oz of water, or fresh fruit or vegetable juice
2 dates (optional if the berries are on the sour side)

Blend together in a blender and serve.

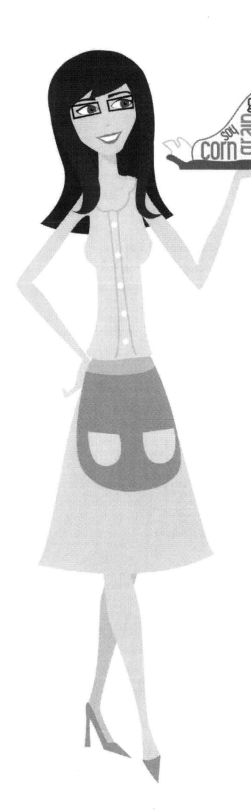

Quality Foods

Good Fats
Pastured Animal Foods

Main Courses/Meat Recipe

Pasture-Raised Animal Foods and Fats

Essential Fatty Acids

- Important for hormone balance
- Formation and fluidity of the cell membrane
- Helps with blood sugar regulation
- Important for the process of creating energy in the cell and helps burn fat
- Brain development and brain function

Omega 3	Omega 6	Omega 9	Saturated Fat
Fish/Fish oil	Borage oil (GLA)	Olive oil	Animal fats
Flax seed oil	Evening primrose oil (GLA)	Avocado	Coconut oil
	Black currant oil (GLA)	Nuts/seeds	Red palm oil
	Hemp seeds/oil (GLA)		
	Nuts/seeds and vegetable oil (veg. not preferred)		

The Vital Roles of Saturated Fat

- **Cell Membranes** – should be 50% saturated fatty acids—main type of fat in brain cells.
- **Bones** – Saturated fats help the body put calcium in the bones—makes strong bones.
- **Heart Function** – Saturated fats are the preferred food for the heart—athletic performance, endurance.
- **Liver** – Saturated fats protect the liver from alcohol & other poisons
- **Lungs** – Can't function without saturated fats—protects against asthma
- **Kidneys** – Can't function without saturated fats
- **Immune System** – Enhanced by saturated fats—fights infection
- **Essential Fatty Acids** – Work together with saturated fats—needed for brain function, healthy skin

Key Nutrients for Brain Development

- **Vitamin A** - Cod liver oil; liver, butter and egg yolks from grass-fed animals
- **Vitamin D** - Cod liver oil; lard, butter and egg yolks from grass-fed animals
- **Choline** - Cod liver oil, egg yolks
- **DHA** - Cod liver oil; liver, butter, egg yolks from grass-fed animals
- **Zinc** - Red meat from grass-fed animals, shellfish
- **Tryptophan** - Meat of grass-fed animals
- **Cholesterol** - Dairy foods, eggs, seafood, meat of grass-fed animals

Recipes that include good fats are listed throughout book.
Some raw coconut oil/butter and avocado recipes in dessert section.

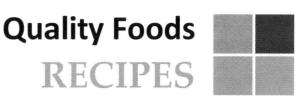

Quality Foods
RECIPES

Sources of Pastured (Not Pasteurized) Foods

California Bay Area Sources

Pastured eggs: Eatwell Farm's Three Wise Hens, Marin Sun Farms, Clark Summit Farms
Pastured raw milk: Organic Pastures, Claravale
Pastured pasteurized milk: Strauss Farms
Pastured/Grass-fed beef: Marin Sun Farms
Pastured/Grass-fed chickens: Hoffman chickens, Marin Sun Farms
High quality organ meats and pates: The Fatted Calf

Pastured – means animals graze on pasture (grass-fed) eating their natural diet of grass (cows) and bugs (chickens) and get plenty of sunlight for adequate vitamin D.
Free-range is NOT pastured.

For sources out of San Francisco, try the Weston A Price Foundation at WestonAPrice.org and connect with a local chapter near you.

Squash Meatballs
GFCF/ SCD/GAPS/Paleo /LOD/FG/FS, Nut-free

To make SCD/Gaps/Paleo, use nut flour in place of GF breadcrumbs. For LOD, use coconut flour. To make nut-free, use a nut-free flour such as coconut flour or GF breadcrumbs. To make this FG, make it without almond flour, and FS without nut flours.

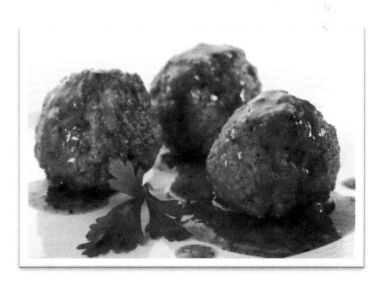

Ingredients
2 lbs ground raw meat (beef, turkey, chicken, buffalo), pastured when possible
1 cups cooked and pureed winter squash (butternut or acorn)
2 eggs
1 cup gluten-free bread crumbs (dry out a few slices of gluten
free bread in oven, crumble by hand or in blender)
Salt to taste (approx. 1 teaspoon)

Directions
1. Preheat the oven to 350 degrees
2. Combine all ingredients. Form into balls and place on parchment paper on baking sheet.
3. Bake at 350 degrees for about 30 minutes or until cooked thoroughly.

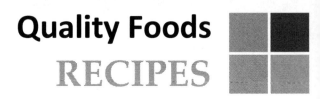

Variation: Puree any vegetables (great way to sneak in vegetables). Over time, you can smash cooked vegetables such as broccoli with a fork instead of pureeing smooth.

This recipe also makes a great meatloaf. Just press into a bread-baking pan and cook at 375 degree for about 1 hour or until thoroughly cooked.

Vegetable Meat Patties
GFCF/ SCD/GAPS/Paleo/LOD/FG/FS, Egg-Free/Nut-Free

Ingredients
1 pound ground meat (any)
1 cup pureed cooked vegetable (any)
1 teaspoon salt

Directions
Mix ground meat, vegetable puree, and salt. Form into patties – you can form these by hand or use a "slider press" from Sur La Table. Heat pan on stove, add cooking oil and cook until thoroughly cooked.

These also make a great a great egg-free meatball.

Chicken Nuggets
GFCF/SCD/GAPS/LOD/FG/FS, Egg-Free/Nut-Free

You can make this SCD with nut flour coating and LOD with coconut flour coating (in place of the first three ingredients). To make nut-free, use a nut-free flour such as coconut flour or GF breadcrumbs. To make it egg-free use a vegetable puree or oil or dairy-free milk to dip before coating breading. To make it FG without almond flour and FS with cashew flour.

Make egg-free by dipping in butternut squash puree instead of eggs.
2 organic chicken breasts with bones removed (use pastured chicken when possible)

Ingredients
Breading choices (choose one)
1 cup GF dry cereal (crushed in a bag)
1 cup GF bread crumbs (dry out bread in oven and crumble in blender)
Almond flour
Any GF or nut flour including coconut flour
1 tablespoons sea salt
2 eggs (or 1 cup of pureed vegetable)

Choose a breading and add salt

Directions

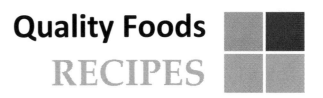
Cut chicken into desired sized strips or pieces, wash and pat dry. Dip chicken into egg or binding mixture, and then coat with breading.

Cook in oil until golden brown.

Egg-Free Chicken Nuggets
GFCF/LOD, Egg-Free/Nut-Free

To make LOD, use LOD allowed flours such as white rice flour.

Ingredients
Chicken breasts or thighs
2/3 cup GF flour (I use 2/3 brown rice flour and 1/3 potato starch or tapioca starch or a combo of both)
2 tsp apple cider vinegar or other GF vinegar
½ tsp baking soda
1/3 cup water
½ tsp salt

Directions
Cut up the chicken into nugget sized pieces.

Measure out your ingredients so you can combine everything fairly rapidly. Mix the flour and salt in the bowl you will use for dipping the chicken. Combine the soda and vinegar and quickly add it to the flour as it fizzes. Quickly add the water next. Mix it together with a fork.

Heat oil in a pan. Dip the chicken in the batter. When the pan is hot enough, place the nuggets in the pan and cook on medium heat. Turn them over half way through cooking so they cook on both sides.

Drain on paper towel. Serve alone or with a dipping sauce. Freeze leftovers.

Chicken Pancakes
GFCF/SCD/GAPS/Paleo/LOD/BED, Nut-Free

Ingredients
1 chicken breast precooked (season as desired while boiling)
3 eggs
½ teaspoon salt

Directions
Blend ingredients together in food processor until completely smooth. Mixture will look like thick pancake batter.

Add a dollop of batter to heated, greased pan and cook like a pancake. Batter may need to be spread out into a pancake shape so it's not too thick.

Egg-Free Chicken Pancakes
GFCF/ SCD/GAPS/Paleo/LOD/BED, Nut-Free, Egg-Free

Ingredients
4 oz ground chicken meat
1 cup pear sauce
¼ teaspoon unrefined salt

Directions
Use ground chicken meat or meat fresh off the bone that you grind or blend in food processor yourself. Place ground meat and pear sauce in food processor and blend until smooth.

Form batter into patties/pancakes. Place in heated, oiled skillet and cook on first side. Cook on low or low-medium, so chicken has plenty of time to cook and firm up before you need to flip. When ready, flip and finish cooking on second side.

Chicken and Squash Flourless Pancakes [Video]
GFCF/ SCD/GAPS/Paleo/LOD/FG/FS, Egg-Free/Nut-Free

Ingredients
½ cup chicken breast, precooked (boiled or roasted)
½ cup squashed, cooked (roasted or steamed)
2 eggs

Directions
Blend ingredients in food processor and cook as pancakes with oil in pan.

Burgers with Liver [Video]
GFCF/ SCD/GAPS/Paleo/LOD/FG, Egg-Free/Nut-Free

Make it FG without herbs and spices except salt.

I know this dish may not sound tasty but these burgers are delicious. No one will know they are eating liver. Liver is a medium oxalate but with the high level of iron, vitamins A & C, zinc, etc., I strongly recommend it.

Ingredients
1 pound ground beef
¼-1/3 cup ground liver

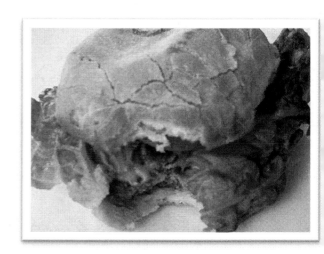

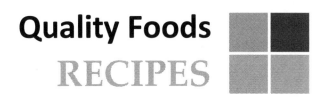
(put liver in food processor and blend until smooth) about 2-3 oz. Avoid any liver that is not thoroughly blended
1-2 teaspoons onion powder
Rosemary, white pepper, or other herb or spice (white pepper is lower oxalate)
Salt, dash

Directions
Mix together and form into patties. Cook as usual – in a pan, on the grill, or as desired.

Chicken Sticks or Cakes
GFCF/SCD/LOD/FG, Nut-Free

Make without spices for FG. These are similar to fish sticks and crab cakes. Use coconut flour instead of nut flour for LOD. You can also use a GF flour instead of a nut flour, depending on dietary needs. You can make this without egg by using 3 Tablespoons of gelatin egg substitute, ½ cup mashed squash (not pureed with water), ½ cup coconut or nut flour (coconut works best).

Ingredients
1 pound chicken, cut up into 1-2 inch chunks or use ground chicken
½ cup onion, finely chopped
1 cup cauliflower (or winter squash)
2 eggs
1 teaspoon thyme
1 teaspoon rosemary
1 teaspoon tarragon
1 teaspoon salt
½ teaspoon pepper (white pepper for LOD)
Oil (ghee or lard) to sauté and pan fry
Extra egg (or puree) to dip in for flour breading
1 cup almond/nut flour

Sauté onions in oil until tender. Add chicken and cook on low until thoroughly cooked, about 20-30 minutes. If any liquid left, drain chicken. To save time you can use roasted chicken from the night before.

Boil cauliflower for 10 minutes while chicken is cooking (or use leftover from night before). You can also use winter squash instead of cauliflower. Drain water from cauliflower and place the cauliflower, chicken, eggs or substitute, herbs, salt and pepper in food processor and blend until finely minced.

Refrigerate mix for 30 minutes until firm and absorb moisture if not sticking together well (should not be too wet). Form into sticks or patties about ½ inch thick and a couple inches long, or into patty shapes. Dip in egg (or puree if avoiding eggs) and then in nut flour.

Pan fry in oil, turning them to brown and cook. Place on paper towel to drain excess oil.
Inspired from "Healing Foods: Cooking for Celiacs, Colitis, Crohn's and IBS" by Sandra Ramacher

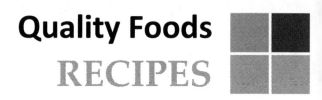

Egg-Free Chicken Patties
GFCF/ SCD/GAPS/Paleo/LOD/BED/FG, Egg-Free/Nut-Free

For LOD, skip the liver.

Ingredients
2 cup of cooked chicken (better boiled than baked)
1/2 cup of cooked cauliflower
¼ cup any other cooked vegetable
¼ onion
1 teaspoon salt
1 garlic clove (optional)
1 cooked chicken liver (optional)
Olive oil or ghee

Directions
Blend the chicken, cauliflower, vegetable, onion, and salt (and optional garlic and liver) together in the food processor. Mixture should be moist enough to and flatten like patties that hold together.
Heat pan and add oil. Pan fry the patties on both sides until browned.

Stir Fry Without Soy Sauce
GFCF/ SCD/GAPS/Paleo/BED/FG, Egg-Free/Nut-Free

Make Feingold (FG) compliant by avoiding red pepper.

Ingredients
1 pound ground meat or cut up meat
2 carrots
1 red pepper
1 stalk of celery
½ onion
1 clove of garlic
1 inch of ginger
6 leaves of greens
1 tablespoon oil (any – sesame is particularly good)
1 tablespoon rice vinegar
Dash of salt

Directions
Add a little oil to a hot pan. Add ginger, garlic and onion, cook for a few minutes on low.

Place meat in pan and cook.

You can do this one of two ways; it partly depends on what vegetables are used. If all fairly quick cooking vegetables are used: peppers, snow peas, greens, celery, etc., cook meat half way through and then add vegetables. When you add the vegetables also add rice vinegar.

If a mixture is used (such as broccoli and carrots, plus peppers and peas), cook meat thoroughly and remove from pan. Cook vegetables separately, starting with the slow cooking vegetable, then add the faster ones so they all turn out even. Remember to add the vinegar when you add the vegetables.

Pot Roast (Dutch oven)
GFCF/SCD/GAPS/Paleo, Nut-Free, Egg-Free

Ingredients
2-3 Lb Chuck Roast (Pasture-raised)
2 Tablespoons cooking fat (ghee, lard, or other oil)
4-5 Carrots peeled and cut in half
1 large onion quartered
3-4 cloves of Garlic halved
2 cups of broth (beef or chicken)
2 teaspoons of dried herbs/spices (my favorite: thyme, rosemary, sage, black pepper, and paprika – any combo)
1 teaspoon sea salt
Splash of wine (optional)

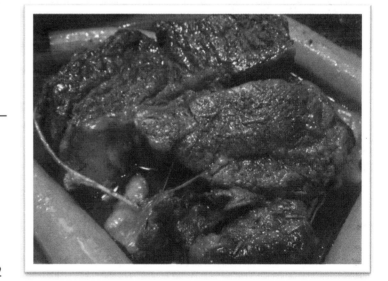

DIrections
Mix herbs/spices and salt together and rub on roast. Heat dutch oven on stove, and add cooking oil. Sear each side of the roast for approximately 2 minutes. Add broth, onion, garlic, and optional splash of wine, and put cover on.

Place in oven at 350 degrees for about 3 to 3 ½ hours. Check every hour to ensure there is enough liquid—to cover the roast about half way. Add water if liquid is getting low. Add the carrots in the last 30 minutes of cooking.

If you don't have a dutch oven, you can also slowly simmer this on the stove or in a crock pot—cooking time will vary based on method.

Salmon Cakes
GFCF/LOD

Ingredients
1, 7.5 oz. wild canned salmon
½ Tablespoon oil (olive, CF ghee melted or other)

2 slices of gluten-free bread (dry out slowly in oven, and then crumble into breadcrumbs)
1 egg
Salt (to taste) – I use canned and salted fish so I add very little extra
½ teaspoon pepper

Directions
Mix ingredients, and let sit for 30 minutes in refrigerator. Form into patties. Heat pan, add oil (ghee or expeller pressed coconut oil), add patties to pan and cook until cooked – several minutes on each side.

Optional: you can add up to 1 cup of finely chopped vegetables like onion, celery, green onion, parsley. Personally, I prefer mine without the vegetables for a more kid-friendly "crab cake" recipe

Salmon Burgers
GFCF/SCD/GAPS/Paleo/FG/LOD

Ingredients
1.5 lbs. skinless, boneless salmon, roughly chopped
2 tsp. parsley
2 tsp. chives
½ teaspoon salt
½ teaspoon pepper (optional)
Olive oil or expeller pressed coconut oil

Directions
Mix the salmon, chives, parsley, salt and pepper together – or toss in food processor. From into patties. Heat pan, add oil and place the patties in pan. Cook for about 10-12 minutes on each side or until done.

Frittata Singles
GFCF/ SCD/GAPS/Paleo/LOD/BED, Nut-free

Potatoes are an optional item in the frittatas for people that don't need to avoid starches.

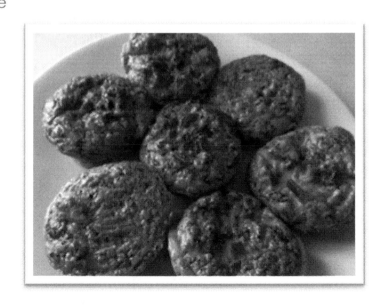

Ingredients

12 pastured eggs
1 ½ cups of raw broccoli, chopped
½ cup red/yellow bell peppers, sliced
1 cup kale, de-stemmed
1 tablespoon fresh chives, chopped
Bacon - 8 pc or 8-12 oz. of bacon
½ teaspoon unrefined salt
½ teaspoon pepper

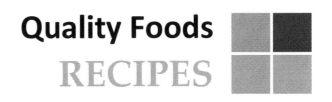

Cook up the bacon on the stove or in the oven, and crumble/cut into pieces. Grease muffin tins. Preheat oven to 350 degrees.

Place all of the vegetables and chives in the food processor and pulse until vegetables are finely chopped, but not pureed/liquefied. Crack eggs in a separate bowl, beat, and add vegetables and bacon.

You can also make one large frittata, rather than singles. My preference with a large frittata is to pour in the egg, and then layer the vegetables and bacon by sprinkling it on the eggs – the vegetables and bacon will sink and you will be able to add the whole vegetable blend.

Pour eggs in muffin cups about 2/3 full.

Bake in the oven at 350 degrees. Frittata singles will take about 25 minutes and one large frittata will take 45 minutes or so. Cook until center is solid.

Deviled Eggs
GFCF, SCD/GAPS/Paleo/LOD, Nut-free

Ingredients
12 eggs (pastured-raised)
1/3 cup mayonnaise (homemade)
1-2 teaspoons Dijon mustard
Sprinkle of salt and pepper

Directions
Garnish with fresh chives, or even salmon roe, if you have it.

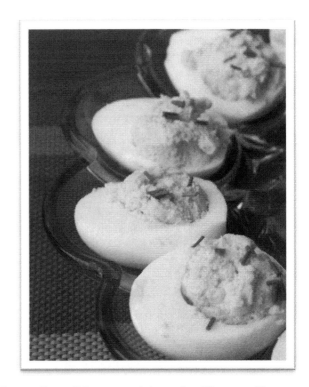

Cook the eggs by hard-boiling them. To do so, fill a pot halfway with water and bring to a gentle boil. Carefully lower eggs one at a time in the water. Set timer for 13 minutes, start timing once you start putting them in the water. Turn up heat until water is boiling again and then adjust heat down to a gentle boil, move eggs around in the pan so that the yolk does not settle to one side. Continue cooking until timer. Do not over cook – yolks will be greenish and sulfur-smelling.

Drain water, and rinse eggs in cold water until pot and water is cool.
Peel eggs. Slice eggs in half. Put yolks into food processor bowl with rest of the ingredients (mayo, mustard, and salt and pepper). Mix in a food processor.

Scoop yolk into white halves. Garnish with chives, salmon eggs, chopped olives, or anything, or serve them plain.

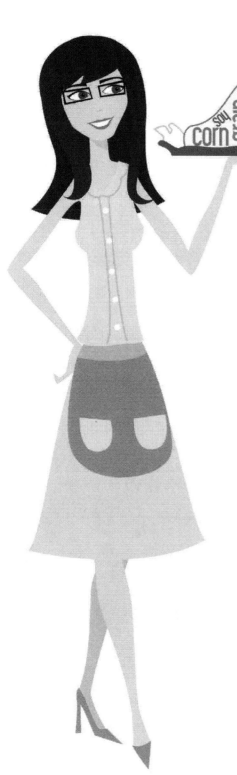

Soaking Seeds & Grains

Milks & Butters
Soaked Bean recipes
Grain-Free Bread/
Baking recipes
Gluten-Free Grain recipes

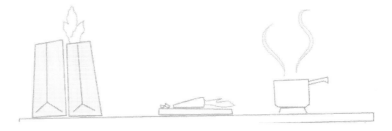

Soaking Seeds & Grains

Enzyme-rich Foods:

Digestible "Seeds" Soaking and Sprouting Grains, Nuts, Seeds, and Beans

It's important to soak, sprout and/or ferment "seeds" – these include grains, beans, and nuts/seeds. Soaking increases the enzyme content, digestibility, and increases nutrient content. This is why I believe so many people have trouble with gluten, soy, and other grains—they are indigestible (or very difficult to digest) without this important process that is missing from modern food processing and home preparation. Grains are one of the most problematic foods for many. One obvious reason for this is that is without proper "processing," grains are difficult to digest because nature created them with special enzyme and nutrient inhibitors.

Phytic acid and oxalates are present on the surface of all seeds, which blocks mineral absorption in the gut, particularly zinc, calcium, magnesium, and iron. Additionally, phytic acid can negatively affect brain function. Interestingly, soy is very high in phytic acid making it very difficult to digest. In Asia they traditionally soak and ferment soy for weeks, if not months.

Instead of needing to break these substances down with digestive enzymes, native cultures knew that soaking and fermenting grains and other seeds activated nature's process of breaking down the phytic acid and keeping people healthy. Soaking seeds in a moist, slightly acidic and warm environment mimics the seeds natural germination process in the soil. When the phytic acid is broken down, the seed can release its enzymes and nutrients for growth. Oxalate levels decrease when seeds are soaked.

Depending on the seed, there are various ways to do this. While it does take some forethought, the process is quite simple and the time commitment minimal. I often use a couple tablespoons of whey in the water to cover the grain in order to create an acidic environment to ferment grains, particularly oats and wheat. Those with casein sensitivity can use lemon juice to create a similar acidity. Additionally, water alone can be used.

One of my favorites is making nut milk this way. While some time and effort is required, by soaking nuts you dramatically increase digestibility and assimilation of nutrients over commercially bought nut milks. You also have more flexibility to make milks with other nuts/seeds to support rotation diets and for those sensitive to the standard almond milk. There is also more "life force" energy in fresh food than boxed food. For example, making your nut milk vs. buying it will greatly increase the digestibility of the milk and the nutrients and energy available in the beverage. Choose what you make based on the diet and time available. If you have the time, it will be worth the wait.

Additionally, raw foods (vegetables, fruits, raw cultured foods) are rich in enzymes and raw foodists swear by this way of eating. While some raw foods are very good, a diet of only raw foods cannot only be difficult to follow but also difficult on the body's digestion. Often those with compromised digestion have difficulty digesting raw foods (as cooking is a form of pre-digestion), and certain vegetables are not supposed to be eaten raw, like cruciferous vegetables and spinach. These are also not recommended in traditional Chinese medicine for pregnant women. Soaking nuts, grains, and beans is a very easy way to have a big impact on digestion and assimilation of nutrients. In the case of grains and beans, when you cook them after soaking, the digestibility is increased. As it also

Soaking Seeds & Grains

decreases cooking time and is fast and easy to do, I think everyone would benefit from this.

Soaking Nuts

Soak nuts such as almonds, walnuts, or pecans in water (with a pinch of salt for flavor if desired). Soak for 7-12 hours. Use almonds for BED compliant recipes.

Soaking Beans

2 cups beans (white, black, kidney, pinto, or black-eyed)

Cover beans with warm water. Add a hearty pinch of baking soda and leave in a warm place for 12-24 hours. Drain, rinse, place in a large pot and add water to cover beans. Bring to a boil and skim off foam. Simmer, covered for 30-60 minutes or until cooked (beans cook much faster when soaked). Don't add salt until finished cooking. Slow cookers also make beans with a wonderful texture—firm and whole but soft and digestible.

Soaking Grains

When soaking grains, place in warm water for 7-24 hour with 2 tablespoons of whey, lemon juice, or vinegar. Drain water and cook with fresh water. Cooks in about 1/3 the time.

Different grains have slightly different amount of whey/lemon juice and soaking times.

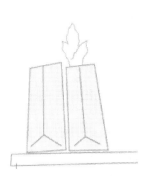

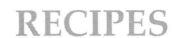

Milks & Butters

Nut Milk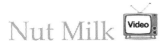
GFCF/ SCD/GAPS/Paleo, FG, Egg-Free

For FG, use nuts other than almonds. Honey for SCD/GAPS/Paleo or no sweetener.

Ingredients
1 C nuts/seeds (any)
Filtered water for soaking nuts
3 C filtered water
Gluten-free vanilla extract
A sweetener - anything you like: a few dates, maple syrup, xylitol, stevia

Directions
I like using almond, cashew, or macadamia nuts. You can also use pine nuts, walnuts, Brazil nuts or anything you like, except peanuts. Soak nuts with a "skin" (such as almonds, pecans or walnuts) overnight. In a hurry, soak nuts for at least 2 hours. For those that are soft with no skin (such as macadamia nuts), no soaking is necessary.

Drain water used to soak nuts.
Combine nuts, fresh water, dates (if used), and blend until creamy.
Strain the milk by pouring the liquid through a vegetable juicer (which strains out the pulp), or with muslin, cheesecloth or thin kitchen towel.
Sweeten and flavor with vanilla and sweetener to taste.
Nut milk will keep two to three days in the refrigerator (no longer). You can also freeze nut milk immediately after making, and thaw as needed.

Cashew Milk
GFCF/ SCD/GAPS/ Paleo/FG, Egg-Free

For cashew milk, the milk does not need to be strained like other nut milks.

Ingredients
1 cup raw cashews, soaked
4 cups of fresh water
1 teaspoon gluten-free vanilla (optional)
1-2 teaspoons raw honey (or other sweetener) (optional)

Soak cashews for at least 2 hours or overnight. Drain cashews and rinse well. Blend all ingredients in the blender.

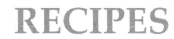

With a standard blender, if you want smoother milk, strain like other nut milks. With a Vitamix, you do not need to strain.

Seed Milk
GFCF/ SCD/GAPS/Paleo/LOD/FG, Egg-Free/Nut-Free

Hemp seeds are not SCD compliant. For LOD, use pumpkin seeds or sunflower seeds. The oxalate level of hemp seeds is unknown at this time.

Ingredients
1 C shelled seeds (pumpkin, sunflower, or hemp)
Filtered water for soaking
3 C filtered water
Gluten-free vanilla extract
1-2 teaspoons of raw honey or other sweetener

Directions
Soak seeds overnight. Drain off water used to soak.

Combine seeds, fresh water, dates (if used) and blend until creamy. Strain the milk. Hemp milk, like cashew milk, is not always strained. Sweeten and flavor with vanilla and sweetener to taste.

Coconut Milk – Dried Coconut
GFCF/ SCD/GAPS/Paleo/LOD/FG, Egg-Free/Nut-Free

Ingredients
1 cup shredded coconut
Boiling water for soaking
1-2 teaspoons of raw honey (optional)

Directions
Place coconut in bowl. Pour boiling or very hot water over coconut. Cover and allow to steep for 30 minutes.
Place coconut and water into blender and blend on high.
Strain the milk.
Sweeten if desired.

Cashew Cream
GFCF/ SCD/GAPS/Paleo/FG/FS, Egg-Free

Ingredients
1 cup raw cashew pieces
1 cup water

Cooking to Heal

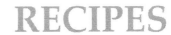

Directions

Cashews can be soaked for a varying amount of time. They soften in 15-20 minutes; however, some people prefer to soak them in water for 6-8 hours, then drain off water. For the purpose of this recipe, cashew cream can also be made when they are not soaked at all.

Blend cashew pieces and water in a blender or food processor until thick and creamy.

Use cashew cream in recipes when a heavy cream texture is desired. Ideal for an ice "cream" recipe. Continue to whip and it will resemble whipped cream.

Hemp Cream
GFCF/Paleo/FG, Nut-Free

Hemp cream is a good alternative for people that can tolerate seeds who are looking for a nut-free "cream."

Ingredients
1 cup raw hemp seeds (hulled)
1 cup water

Directions

Like cashew cream, for the purpose of this recipe, the hemp seeds can be soaked or not soaked. For those looking for the digestive benefits of soaking, soak hemp seeds in water for 6-8 hours. Drain off water.

Blend hemp seeds and water in a blender or food processor until thick and creamy.

Coconut Whipped Cream
GFCF/SCD/GAPS/Paleo/LOD/FG, Egg-free and Nut-free

Use honey as the sweetener for SCD/GAPS. Wilderness Family Naturals makes a great coconut cream.

Ingredients
8 oz of coconut cream, chilled for 30 minutes in refrigerator (or two cans of coconut milk).
½ teaspoon vanilla extract (GF)
1 tablespoon of sweetener of your choice (honey, cane sugar, or other)

Directions

If you have cans of coconut milk, chill the cans for 30 minutes. Then open the cans and scoop solid/thick part of coconut into a bowl (use liquid in a smoothie or beverage). Continue to chill in bowl for 15 more minutes.

Start with chilled coconut cream in a bowl, add vanilla, and sweetener. Beat with electric whisk or mixer, until whipped into peaks. If you desire more firm peaks, place bowl of cream in refrigerator again for 20-30 minutes. Then whip until finished.

Soaking Seeds & Grains
RECIPES

Rice/Oat Milk
GFCF/LOD/FG/FS, Egg-Free/Nut-Free

For LOD, use rice. White rice has lowest oxalate content but also the least nutrients. For oat milk, you must use oats that are certified gluten-free to be sure it will not contain any gluten.

Homemade rice milk or oat milk is worth the effort because you can make it unsweetened - to be used in recipes - or with much less sugar than the store brands contain. Also, the store bought varieties may contain carrageenan, a thickener that can be inflammatory to the gut.

Ingredients
1 cup of cooked rice (brown or white) or GF oats (rolled or steel cut)
4 cups warm water
1 teaspoon gluten-free vanilla
1-3 teaspoons of raw honey or maple syrup – sweetened to taste (optional)

Directions
Add grain and water to blender and blend. Strain through nut milk bag or cloth. Sweeten and add vanilla as desired.

Crispy Almonds
GFCF/ SCD/GAPS/Paleo/BED, Egg-Free

Dehydrator helpful.

Ingredients
4 cups raw almonds
sea salt
Filtered water

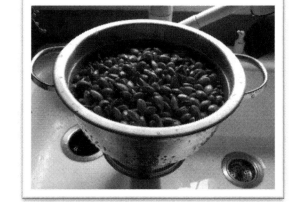

Directions
Rinse nuts. Soak almonds overnight (or for 8 hour). Drain and rinse nuts. Sprinkle salt on nuts, if desired. Dehydrate nuts in a food dehydrator for about 24-36 hours at 115 degrees. Store in an airtight container.

You may also use a warming oven or a regular oven at the lowest temperature possible; however, the higher the temperature, the more roasted they will be and they will lose some fatty acid benefits.

Spread nuts on a baking pan at the lowest temperature possible. Cooking time will range from a couple hours up to 24 hours.

Nuts are done once they are completely dry—when you bite into one, it should be crispy and not soggy at all.

Soaking Seeds & Grains
RECIPES

Crispy Nuts
GFCF/ SCD/GAPS/Paleo/BED, Egg-Free

Try walnuts and pecans using the crispy almond recipe. Soak walnuts for 4 hours, and pecans for 6 hours.

Crispy Seeds
GFCF/ SCD/GAPS/Paleo/LOD/BED, Nut-Free/Egg-Free

Follow the Crispy Almond recipe with pumpkin and/or sunflower seeds.

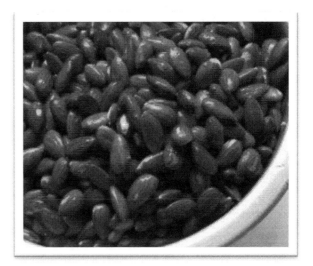

Roasted Pumpkin Seeds
GFCF/SCD/GAPS/Paleo/LOD, Nut-Free, Egg-Free

For lower oxalate, avoid high oxalate spices.

Ingredients
3 cups pumpkin seeds (soak for 8 hours)
2 T extra virgin olive oil
½ to 1 teaspoon unrefined sea salt
Herbs or spices (optional) – I like 1 teaspoon ground turmeric powder, 1 teaspoon ground ginger powder and ¼ teaspoon cardamom.

Directions
Drain and rinse soaked pumpkin seeds and place in a bowl. Add the olive oil and mix to coat. Sprinkle on spices and salt and mix. Spread a thin layer of seeds on several cookie sheets.

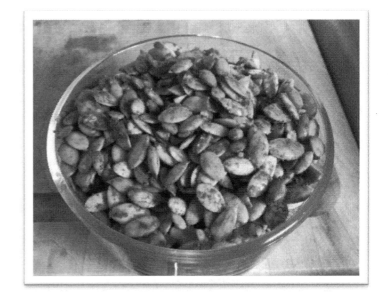

Either bake or dehydrate. To bake, put on 200 degrees for approximately 45 minutes. However, check them at 10 minutes to make sure your oven isn't too hot. Try not to brown them.   To dehydrate: place the seeds on the dehydrator sheets, place in dehydrator at 110 degrees for about 24 hours. They are done when they are no longer wet / moist at all, and instead are crispy.

Inspired by Trudy Scott, author of *The Anti-Anxiety Food Solution*.

Snack Mix
GFCF/ SCD/Gaps/Paleo, Nut-Free and Egg-Free

Ingredients
Salted crispy seeds
Crispy kale
Carrot chips

Directions
Combine crispy seeds, crispy kale, and carrot chips together and serve as a snack. You can also add other vegetable chips

Nut Butter
GFCF/ SCD/GAPS/Paleo/FG/FS, Egg-Free

To make FG, use nuts other than almonds and no honey. FS make only with cashews and sunflower oil, and no honey.

Ingredients
2 cups soaked and dried nuts ("crispy nuts")
1/3 cup raw coconut oil
1/3 cup nut/seed oil such as pumpkinseed oil
½-1 Tablespoon raw honey
¼ - ½ sea salt

Directions
Place nuts in food processor and grind to a powder. Add oils and blend until smooth. Slowly add salt and honey a little at a time until desired flavor is reached. You can adjust the amount of coconut and pumpkinseed oil to get desired texture. While it will start out soft, coconut oil gets very hard in the refrigerator—over time you will determine the right texture your child will like.

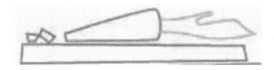

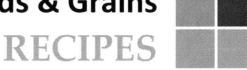
Soaked Bean Dishes

Yellow Lentil Pancakes (Moong Dal Chila)
GFCF/ SCD/GAPS/LOD/FG, Egg-Free/Nut-Free

These are traditional Indian pancakes made with moong dal – a type of split yellow mung bean that has been skinned. You will most likely need to find these at an Indian store. You may try making them with other types of lentils that are more easily found at the store (although I haven't tried this). These pancakes are great because they are egg-free.

Ingredients
Lentils, 1 cup
Water
Oil
Salt

Directions
Soak lentils in water on counter overnight. Drain water and grind to a smooth paste. Add enough water to make a pancake batter.

Add 1-2 teaspoons oil to a pan for cooking pancakes. Drop batter into pan and cook like pancakes.

Dosas (Fermented Lentil/Rice Pancakes)
GFCF/LOD, Egg-Free/Nut-Free

Fermenting grains and legumes allows for lectins (inflammatory compounds) and proteins to breakdown for better digestion.

Ingredients
2 cups white rice
2/3 cup urad dal (Indian split lentils)
½ teaspoon fenugreek seeds
½ cup water
½ teaspoon salt
oil

Directions
Put rice in one bowl and lentils and fenugreek seeds in the other. Soak both in enough water that it covers by 2 inches overnight.

Next day, drain and grind the rice and lentils separately in a blender and blend smooth adding just enough water (up to ¼ cup) to end up with a fairly thick batter. In a larger bowl, mix the batters together and add the salt. Cover and place in a warm, dry spot. Allow it to ferment on the counter until fluffy with tiny bubbles. This will take at least 24 hours.

After fermentation, add enough water whipping it together with a fork to make it fluffier—making the batter thick but pourable.

Cook as you would pancakes by heating an iron skillet or pan. Add a bit of oil to the hot pan and pour batter with a ladle then spread the batter out slightly to make a thin pancake. Cooking until golden brown.

Serve plain, with a spread, or fill with vegetables/meats.

From "1,000 Indian Recipes" by Neelam Batra – I highly recommend this book!

Roasted Garbanzo Bean Snack
GFCF, Egg-Free/Nut-Free

This recipe uses cooked beans—read entire recipe before beginning.

Ingredients
3 cups garbanzo beans, cooked* (firm not soft)
1 tablespoon maple syrup
1 Tablespoons oil such as olive oil
1/2 teaspoon salt
Herbs and spices (some combinations: ½ teaspoon of cinnamon, cardamom, and cumin; any combination of herbs and spices, or plain with salt only)

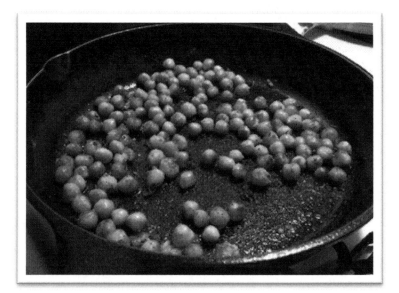

Directions
While homemade cooked beans are better for you and more easily digestible, you can use canned beans in a pinch. Rinse well and drain. If you are cooking beans yourself: Soak beans for 8-12 hours in water. Drain water. Rinse beans. Cook in a pot with fresh water until cooked but still firm, or use the slow cooker. Do not allow beans to overcook.

In a large bowl, toss together beans and all remaining ingredients including the oil. Let "marinate" for 15 minutes.

While you can cook these in the oven, I prefer an iron skillet on the stovetop. Spread beans out into a single layer on a heated, oiled skillet.

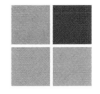
Heat pan to medium/high, stir occasionally. Roast them on stovetop for 30-45 minutes, depending how dry and crunchy you want them. You can also finish by dehydrating them if you want them very dry and crispy – they store best this way

Bean Burgers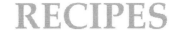
GFCF/ SCD/GAPS/FG, Nut-Free

To make FG, limit herbs and spices to parsley, salt and pepper.

Ingredients

1 cup black or kidney beans
1 cup sunflower seeds
4 eggs
½ cup carrots – peeled, grated
½ cup kale – finely chopped
½ cup onion – finely chopped
1 Tablespoon fresh parsley – finely chopped
1 Tablespoon rosemary
1 Tablespoon basil
1 ¼ teaspoons salt
Pepper (optional)
Ghee, lard, or expeller-pressed coconut oil to use for cooking.

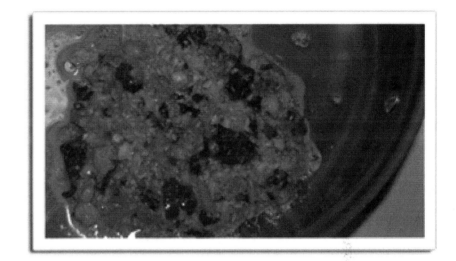

Directions

Soak the beans overnight in water with a pinch of baking soda. Drain and rinse with water. Place the beans into a pot and cover with water and cook for 20-25 minutes until soft, but not mushy. Do not add salt to the beans while they cook—it will make them tough.

Grind the sunflower seeds until the consistency of nut flour. Place beans into a food processor and process until coarsely chopped. Combine with the sunflower seed meal, carrots, kale, onion, herbs, eggs, salt, and pepper, and knead with your hands until mixed thoroughly. Form into patties and fry in a skillet with the oil. Cook on medium for at least 10 minutes on each side. These burgers can be kept from up to 3 days, They can be eaten cold or reheated in the over on 340 degrees for about 10 minutes. They will also freeze well. Makes 10 burgers.

LOD Bean Burgers
GFCF/LOD/FG, Nut-Free

To make FG, limit herbs and spices to parsley, salt and pepper, and use zucchini only if tolerated (otherwise, use a different vegetable).

Black-eyed peas are not SCD/Gaps compliant, but are LOD.

Ingredients
1 cup black-eyed peas
1 cup pumpkin seeds
4 eggs
½ cup zucchini –grated
½ cup onion – finely chopped
1 Tablespoon basil
1 Tablespoon sage
1 teaspoon unrefined salt (be generous) and white pepper

Directions
Ghee or coconut oil to cook in.

Soak the black-eyed peas overnight with water and a pinch of baking soda.

Grind the seeds until the consistency of nut flour. Place peas into a food processor and process until coarsely chopped. Combine with the seed meal, zucchini, onion, herbs, eggs, and salt, and knead with your hands until mixed thoroughly. Form into patties and fry in a skillet with the oil. Cook on medium for at least 10 minutes on each side. These burgers can be kept from up to 3 days, They can be eaten cold or reheated in the over on 340 degrees for about 10 minutes. They will also freeze well. Makes 10 burgers.

Egg-Free Bean Burgers with Rice
GFCF/LOD/FG, Nut-Free

For low oxalates beans, lentils or peas.

Ingredients
1 cup cooked beans (soaked and cooked beans)
1 cup cooked rice
1 cup ground sunflower seeds
1 cup grated carrots
½ teaspoon salt

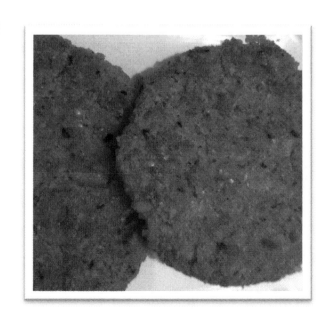

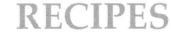

Directions
First, grind sunflower seeds in food processor into a flour, add carrots and process. Finally, add beans and rice and pulse until mixed.

Form into patties and panfry in oil (any, expeller pressed coconut or ghee are my favorites) until thoroughly heated. Serve with lettuce wrap or a bun.

Boston Baked Beans
GFCF/GAPS, Nut-Free, Egg-Free

Use honey for GAPS diet. This is recipe is not too sweet.

Ingredients
4 cups dry navy (white) beans (1.5 pounds or 725 grams) –
Soak beans in water overnight in a bowl on the counter)
1 bay leaf
¼-½ cup blackstrap molasses
1 ½ Tablespoons onion powder (or 1 chopped onion –
consider whether your child likes chunks of onion, if not
use dried powder)
1 teaspoon dry mustard powder
2 teaspoons sea salt
½ teaspoon ground pepper (optional)
½ lb of bacon, cut into pieces (optional)
After 8 hours of soaking beans, drain and rinse beans.

Directions
Preheat oven to 350 degrees F.

Place beans in pot covered with fresh water, add 1 bay leaf. Bring to a boil, then reduce to a simmer for 10 minutes, skim off foam and dump. Drain beans and reserve liquid. You can either reuse liquid or use fresh water – fresh water makes for more digestible beans.

Place beans in Dutch oven, add all of the ingredients, stir, and add enough liquid to just cover beans (either reserve liquid or fresh water). Cover Dutch oven and cook in oven for 2 hours – check half way through to make sure the beans are not drying out. If the water level goes below the beans, they will dry out instead of softening and cooking properly. Add more water if the level drops.

Once beans begin to get tender (about 2 hours), remove cover and cook for 30 more minutes. This will evaporate some of the liquid making the sauce thicker. You can also blend 1 cup of beans with 1 cup of liquid, and add back to beans for a thickened sauce.

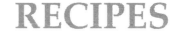
Garbanzo and Squash Stew
GFCF/LOD, Egg-Free/Nut-Free

To make this recipe LOD, substitute ½ bunch of collard greens or other vegetable for the kale, and use acorn as the squash.

Soak and cook beans ahead of time. I cook my beans in a slow cooker with plenty of water covering them, for 5 ½ hours on low, this way I don't have to watch the pot and the beans are firmer and less water logged.

Ingredients
½ lb bacon (pan fried, save bacon grease)
2 Tablespoons bacon fat (from cooking bacon)
½ onion, finely chopped
3 cloves garlic (minced or crushed)
1 ½ cups of diced tomatoes
2-3 squash (depending on size) – You can use acorn, butternut, kabocha, or delicata (delicata is great because the skin is soft and edible, so you don't need to peel them.
1 teaspoon garam masala (optional)
1 bunch kale, finely chopped
4 cups cooked garbanzo beans
1 cup of water or chicken stock
1 teaspoon of salt

Directions
Saute onions in bacon fat on medium heat for about 3-5 minutes. Add garlic and tomato, sauté briefly (a minute or so). Add squash and garam masala, bring to a simmer and cook on low until squash is tender but not too soft (about 15 minutes). Add cooked beans, water or stock, and salt. Simmer for an additional 5 minutes.

Grain-Free Bread / Baking

Light White Bread – 1 Loaf
GFCF/SCD/Gaps

Ingredients
2 ½ cups almond flour
1 tsp baking soda
¼ tsp salt
3 eggs – separated
1 cup nut milk yogurt
1 Tablespoon honey

Directions
Preheat oven to 300 degrees
Line 4 x 8 inch loaf tin with parchment paper

In a large bowl, mix the almond flour, baking soda and salt. Whisk the egg yolks with the yogurt and honey until light and fluffy. Beat the egg whites until stiff. Combine the egg yolk mixture with the almond flour until smooth. Add the stiff egg whites and gently blend. Pour the mixture into the prepared loaf tin and bake for 50-60 minutes or until the top feels spongy. Let cool before slicing. Refrigerate in an airtight container.

This is soft and fluffy bread, great with savory or sweet toppings. It is too soft for the toaster, but will toast nicely under the grill.

Adapted from "Healing Foods: Cooking for Celiacs, Colitis, Crohn's and IBS" by Sandra Ramacher

Cashew Butter Bread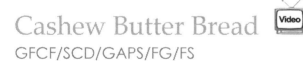
GFCF/SCD/GAPS/FG/FS

Ingredients
3 eggs
1 1/4 cups cashew butter
½ cup nut milk
1 teaspoon honey (honey is not FG or FS, eliminate or use another sweetener for these diets)
1 teaspoon baking soda
1 teaspoon salt

Directions
Heat oven to 325 degrees. Line loaf pan with parchment paper.

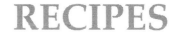

Mix eggs, cashew butter, nut milk, honey, baking soda and salt. Pour into prepared pan.

Bake for 30-40 minutes

Nut Butter Pancake
GFCF/ SCD/GAPS/ FG, Nut-Free

Can be made nut-free with sunflower seed butter.

Ingredients
1 tablespoon nut or seed butter
1 egg
¼ teaspoon of baking soda
Ghee for pan

Directions
In a bowl, beat egg well with a fork.   Add nut/seed butter and baking soda and mix by hand until well blended. Heat pan, then add ghee to coat pan. Scoop batter into pan and cook as you would any pancake. Make sure heat is not too high (medium/low) so pancake has a chance to cook and set before turning (and burning). Flip pancake, and cook second side. Best topped with honey.

Coconut Pancakes (Grain-Free)
GFCF/SCD/GAPS/ LOD, Nut-free

Ingredients
1/4 cup, (plus 1 Tablespoon) coconut flour
¼ teaspoon unrefined salt
1/4 teaspoon baking soda
4 large or 5 medium pastured eggs (room temperature)
2 Tablespoons of non-dairy milk (room temperature)
1 teaspoon vanilla extract
1/4 cup melted coconut oil or ghee
½ Tablespoon raw honey (or other sweetner if not on SCD) – sweetener is optional

Directions
Beat eggs in large bowl; add non-dairy milk, honey, vanilla, and ¼ cup melted oil. In a separate bowl combine ¼ cup coconut flour, salt, baking soda—next, place this flour blend in sifter. Sift flour into liquids bowl little by little while mixing it with an electric mixer until combined and smooth. If pancake batter is too thin add 1 Tablespoon of coconut flour. If it's too think to pour or scoop, thin with more non-dairy milk.

Scoop batter into hot, oiled skillet (use unflavored coconut). Cook at low-medium temperature. Flip when ready and cook on second side

Banana Pancakes (with Coconut Flour Blend)
GFCF/LOD/FG, Nut-Free

Ingredients
1 cup rice flour (white or brown)
1/3 cup coconut flour
2 T potato starch or tapioca starch
2 teaspoon baking powder
1 tablespoon sugar
4 eggs
2 bananas
2 tablespoons oil (melted coconut or any)
1 ½ cup non-dairy milk

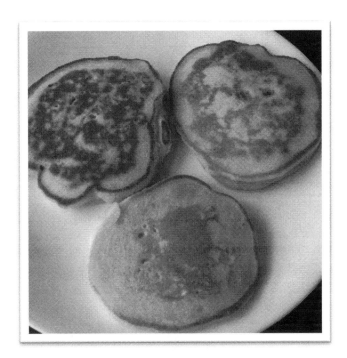

Directions
Beat eggs, then mash in bananas, add oil and non-dairy milk. In a separate bowl combine all dry ingredients. Sift (if you have a sifter) flour/dry ingredient blend into wet ingredients gradually while mixing with an electric mixer or by hand. Add more liquid if too thick.

Pour batter into hot, oiled pan and cook pancakes over low/medium heat. Then flip and serve when done. Makes 12-14 pancakes

Grain-Free Herb Crackers
GFCF/SCD/Gaps

Ingredients
1 loaf Cashew Butter Bread, thinly sliced
½ cup ghee
1-2 cloves of garlic, minced
1-2 teaspoon herb (Italian mix of oregano and basil, rosemary, or any combination)
Unrefined Salt

Directions
Melt ghee, add minced garlic and herbs- and mix around to incorporate flavors into ghee – let sit for 15 minutes. Brush ghee mixture on both sides of bread. Sprinkle salt on each piece.

Either baked these in the oven at the lowest temperature possible for several hours, or dehydrate these in a dehydrator at 150 degrees for 8 hours. Place in airtight container.

Grain-Free Cereal
GFCF/ SCD/Gaps

Ingredients
3 Tablespoons ghee
1 -2 Tablespoons honey
¼ teaspoon gluten-free vanilla
a tiny dash of cinnamon to taste (about 1/16 of a teaspoon)

Directions
This is a spin off of the Herb Crackers. Thinly slice the light white or cashew bread. "Butter" each side of the bread with the honey and ghee mixture with a pastry brush. Cut into small centimeter sized bites (cereal size) and dehydrate at 150°F for eight hours.

Great as a dry snack or with milk (dairy-free of course).

Cashew Butter Tortillas
GFCF/ SCD/GAPS/FG

Ingredients
2 cups raw cashew butter
3 eggs
2 Tablespoons ghee, melted
1/2 freshly squeezed lemon or lime juice
1 teaspoon salt
½ teaspoon baking soda
3 cups fresh water

Directions
In a food processor, puree the cashew butter, eggs, ghee, lemon/lime juice, salt, and baking soda until smooth. Add water and blend smooth.

Heat skillet and Pour thin batter into a hot skillet. Place parchment paper between each tortilla, so they won't stick together. Store in a plastic bag in the refrigerator for a week or in the freezer.

Banana-Coconut Bread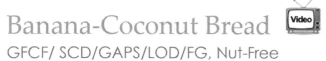
GFCF/ SCD/GAPS/LOD/FG, Nut-Free

To make FG, use sweetener other than honey such as maple syrup (maple is not SCD/Gaps compliant).

Ingredients
4 ripe bananas with brown spots (pureed in food processor with no liquid)

6 eggs
1/3 cup coconut oil (melted)
1/2 cup honey
1 Tablespoon lemon juice
1 teaspoon gluten-free vanilla extract
1 cup pumpkin seed flour (grind pumpkin seeds)
1 cup coconut flour
2 teaspoons baking soda

Directions
Preheat oven to 350 degrees. Mix pureed bananas, eggs, melted coconut oil, honey, lemon juice, and vanilla.

Grind pumpkinseeds in food processor until coarse flour-like consistency. Hungarian pumpkin seeds are less oily and make great flour.

Add dry ingredients. Spread in greased pan. Bake approximately 45-50 minutes.

Crispy Chickpea Flour Pancakes
GFCF, Egg-Free/Nut-Free

This is an adaptation of an Indian recipe. Made with chickpea (garbanzo bean) flour. While you can buy chickpea flour (it can be a bit hard to find), you can also make with dried peas using a Vitamix and the grain attachment or a grain flourmill.

These can be made with or without the hot peppers. While they may make it too spicy for children or be difficult with digestive disturbances, many adults find the peppers a delicious addition.   Include them or eliminate them based on your needs.

Ingredients
2 cups chickpea flour
1 onion (finely minced)
1 ½ tablespoon fresh peeled ginger (finely minced)
½ cup fresh cilantro (finely chopped)
1-3 fresh green chili peppers (finely minced with seeds)
1 tablespoon ground coriander
1 ½ teaspoons salt
½ teaspoon baking soda
1 ½ to 2 cups of water
oil

Directions

Mix everything together except the water and oil. Add the water to make a batter of pourable consistency (medium thickness). Whip with a fork to make it fluffy. Set aside for 30 minutes—the batter will continue to thicken.

Heat iron skillet or pan and add a bit oil to cook. Cook as you would pancakes. Add a bit of oil to the hot pan and pour batter with a ladle then spread the batter out slightly to make a thin pancake. Cook until golden brown.

Serve plain or with a "yogurt" sauce. Yogurt sauce can be made with non-dairy yogurt, cashew cream, or homemade yogurt (if allowed).

Chickpea Pancakes
GFCF, Egg-Free/Nut-Free

These are just like the Chickpea Flour Pancakes but made with soaked chickpeas (garbanzo bean) instead of pea flour. Soaked whole beans/peas are easier to find and more digestible.

Just like the others, these can be made with or without the hot peppers. While they may make it too spicy for children or be difficult with digestive disturbances, many adults find the peppers a delicious addition.   Include them or eliminate them based on your needs.

Ingredients
2 ½ to 3 cups garbanzo beans (soaked for 8 hours, drained and well rinsed)
1 onion (finely minced)
1 ½ tablespoon fresh peeled ginger (finely minced)
½ cup fresh cilantro (finely chopped)
1-3 fresh green chili peppers (finely minced with seeds)
1 tablespoon ground coriander
1 ½ teaspoons salt
½ teaspoon baking soda
1 ½ to 2 cups of water
oil

Directions
Blend soaked beans in blender or food processor. Mix everything together except the water and oil. Add the water to make a batter of pourable consistency (medium thickness). Whip with a fork to make it fluffy. Set aside for 30 minutes—the batter will continue to thicken.

Heat iron skillet or pan and add a bit oil to cook. Cook as you would pancakes. Add a bit of oil to the hot pan and pour batter with a ladle then spread the batter out slightly to make a thin pancake. Cooking until golden brown.
Serve plain or with a "yogurt" sauce. Yogurt sauce can be made with non-dairy yogurt, cashew cream, or homemade yogurt (if allowed).

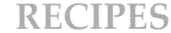

Gluten-Free Grain Recipes

Julie and Carla's Granola
GFCF/FG

This recipe requires fermenting and dehydrating oats ahead of time. To make FG compliant, prepare without almonds or raisins.

Ingredients
16 cups rolled oats (use oats from GlutenFreeOats.com or OnlyOats.com)
1/3-1/2 cup coconut kefir to soak oats
1 cup coconut flakes
4 cups chopped crispy nuts
raisins or dried fruit (as desired)

Wet ingredients
1 cup coconut oil
2/3 cup maple syrup
3-4 Tablespoons brown sugar (optional)
2 teaspoon vanilla extract (gluten-free)
1/2 teaspoon salt

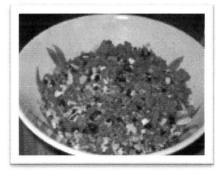

Soak and ferment oats
Soak oats by covering with filtered water and 1/3-1/2 cup coconut kefir (or whey if not casein-free). (You can also try lemon juice but it may be a bit sour and will not "ferment" it. Plain water can be used to soak it too.) Place in warm location and soak for 7-24 hours. Drain oats by pushing a bowl onto oats while in strainer.

Spread fairly thin on dehydrator sheets and dehydrate at 115 degrees until completely dry, about 8-16 hours. I often do this while dehydrating nuts.

Break up dehydrated oats into small clusters in a bowl. Set aside.

Warm up wet ingredients (except vanilla) until runny. (Sugar does not melt.) Remove from heat and add vanilla. Pour into container and whisk as you drizzle over oats. Do not add the nuts, coconut flakes or fruit yet. Oats are the only things coated and baked.

Toast on cookie sheet at 225 degrees for 45 minutes. Stir occasionally. In the last 5 minutes you can add the coconut flakes for a light toasting. Cool oats.

Add chopped crispy nuts and dried fruit. Store in airtight containers. Makes 20-22 cups of granola.

LOD Pancakes Without Eggs
GFCF/LOD/FG, Nut-Free/Egg-Free

To make FG, use pear puree. For LOD, you can use some potato starch and/or other low oxalate flours as a blend, rather than straight white rice flour.

Ingredients
2 cups white rice flour
1 teaspoon baking soda
½ teaspoon salt
1 Tablespoon of vinegar (such as apple cider vinegar)
¼ cup melted ghee or any oil
½ cup pureed LOD fruit such as apple or pear
1 ½ cups water

Directions
Combine flour and salt. In a separate bowl, combine vinegar and baking soda, and then add other wet ingredients (oil, fruit puree, and water). Mix the wet ingredients into the dry ingredients. If the batter is too thick, add a bit more water until desired texture.

Heat pan and then add oil. Cook as you would any pancakes.

Breads From Anna™ - Yeast-Free Bread Mix
GFCF, Nut-Free

Makes yeast-free bread, pizza crust, and buns.

Ingredients
Bread Mix from Breads from Anna
2 Tablespoons oil
1 ½ cups non-dairy milk
2 eggs
1 egg white

Directions
Blend eggs and egg white until creamy. Combine remaining wet ingredients. Slowly add dry ingredients and mix well.   Do not over mix. Place into greased and floured (GF) 8½ x 4 ½ loaf pan. Bake for 70 minutes at 375 degrees.

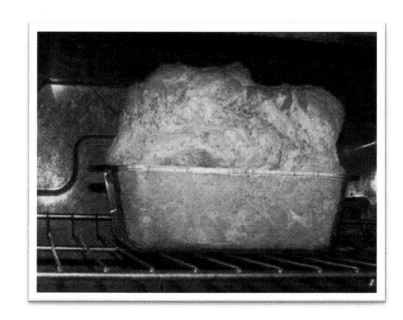

To make pizza or buns, combine ingredients as above, then spread on baking sheet or stoneware into pizza shape, or form into buns.

Mixes available at www.breadsfromanna.com

Unleavened Indian Bread (Chapati)
GFCF, Egg-Free/Nut-Free

This is a gluten-free Chapati. Usually this bread is made with gluten flour. I've found that gluten-free oat flour works well.

Ingredients
2 cups GF oat flour
1 cup water

Directions
Place flour in a bowl and add ¾ cup of water. Mix the flour lightly with your hands. Add more water if too dry and firm, or more flour if too sticky. Knead dough for 1 minute by pressing the dough down with your palm or knuckles, gathering it together into a ball and pressing again. If the dough is pliable—not too sticky and not too firm, it's the right consistency.

Cover dough and let it sit for 1-2 hours.

Form into small balls. Press out by hand on to floured board, adding flour to both sides of dough while pressing. Cook on hot skillet with a bit of ghee on both sides until done.

Rice Porridge (Slow Cooker)
GFCF/ Nut-Free, Egg-Free

Can be made egg-free by eliminating egg – while it will not be quite as thick, it's still delicious.

Similar to rice pudding but less sweet and for breakfast

Ingredients
1 ¼ cup brown rice
1 ½ cups (1 can) coconut milk
1 ½ cups water
1 beaten egg
1 teaspoon vanilla
1 teaspoon cinnamon
½ teaspoon cardamom
¼ teaspoon ginger powder

¼ teaspoon nutmeg
2-3 tablespoons of honey or maple syrup

Directions
Place all ingredients in slow cooker and cook on low for 5 hours. Set timer at night, and breakfast will be ready when you wake up.

If you don't have or want to use a slow cooker, you can combine all of the ingredients in a pot and simmer for 50 minutes or until done.

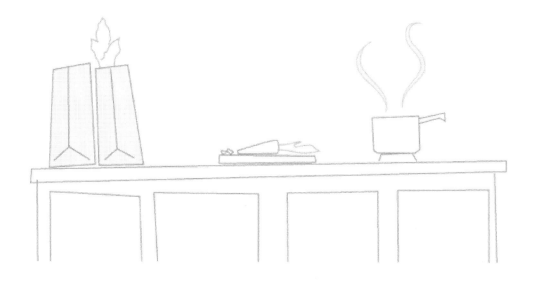

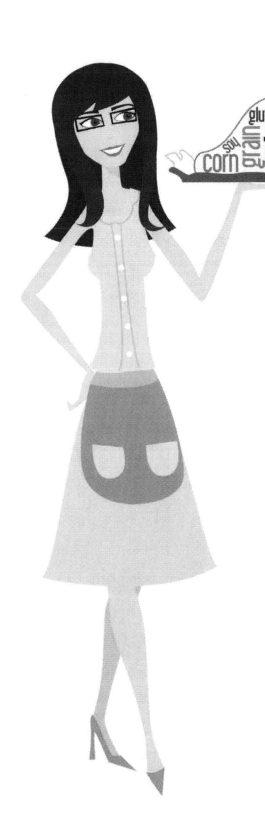

Desserts

Gluten-Free and Grain-Free recipes

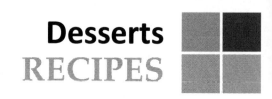

Coconut Date Balls
GFCF/ SCD/GAPS/Paleo/FG, Egg-Free/Nut-Free

Ingredients
1 ½ cups pitted dates
½-3/4 cup coconut butter (sometimes called coconut spread, not the same as coconut oil) or other nut butter
1 tablespoon of raw coconut oil (more if using nut butter not coconut butter)
¼ cup finely shredded dried coconut
1 cup finely shredded dried coconut (used for rolling the balls)

Directions
In a food processor, blend the dates into paste. Add the coconut butter or nut butter and pulse a few times until the ingredients are mixed. If too difficult/sticky to pulse with nut butter, mix by hand. Add dried coconut and process for 5 to 10 seconds more. Melt coconut oil and add to processor. Roll into balls.

Melt additional coconut oil. Coat the ball with oil then roll in shredded coconut.

Store in a cool place, such as the refrigerator.

Coconut Date Ball Variations:

Use coconut butter instead of nut butter (not coconut oil). Sometimes called coconut spread. Found online: wildernessfamilynaturals.com
Use sunflower seed butter instead of nut butter if allergic to nuts (if seeds are allowed)
Add chopped fruit
Add sultanas (raisins)
Add chopped nuts
Roll in sesame seeds
Add GF chocolate chips for a treat
Coat in cocoa powder

Chocolate Chip "Raw Cookie Dough" Balls
GFCF, Egg-Free/Nut-Free

Use the Coconut Date Ball recipe, and add GFCF chocolate chips to batter. Form into balls.

This recipe tastes very similar to raw cookie dough (however, it does not cook up into cookies).

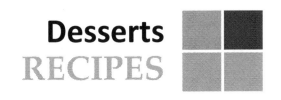

Coconut White Fudge
GFCF/SCD/GAPS/Paleo/LOD/FG, Egg-Free/Nut-Free

Ingredients
1 cup coconut butter
1 teaspoon raw coconut oil
1-2 Tablespoon raw honey (to taste)

If desired, baking extract such as orange extract, gluten-free vanilla extract or citrus oils
Orange or lemon rind (for fruit extracts)

Directions
Add coconut butter to food processor and chop up into fine chunks. Melt coconut oil (not too hot) and add to food processor while spinning. Slowly add honey and extract/rind. Taste as you go to achieve desired sweetness.

Place waxed paper on cookie sheet. Scoop mixture onto paper, and spread thinly (1/3-1/2 inch) and put pan in refrigerator to chill. Take out and cut into small ½ inch squares. Peel off paper and store in airtight container in the refrigerator.

Variations: You can make chocolate fudge by adding unsweetened cocoa powder (ideally organic and fair trade). You will need more honey as the cocoa is bitter. Cocoa is not SCD/Gaps legal.

Cocoa Mints
GFCF/Paleo, Egg-Free/Nut-Free

Ingredients
1½ cup coconut butter
½ teaspoon raw coconut oil
5-8 drops peppermint oil
1-2 Tablespoons raw honey
Unsweetened cocoa powder

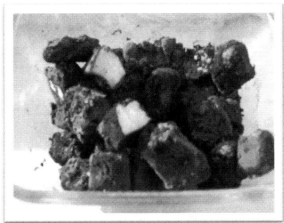

Directions
Add coconut butter to food processor and chop up into fine chunks. Melt coconut oil (not too hot) and add to food processor while spinning. Slowly add honey and peppermint oil and taste as you go to achieve desired sweetness.

Place waxed paper on cookie sheet. Scoop mixture onto paper, and spread 1/2 inch thick, and put pan in refrigerator to chill for 10 minutes. Before too cold and hard, take out of frig and cut into 1/2 inch or smaller squares.

While still a little soft, roll in unsweetened cocoa. If not sticking, roll in a bit of warm (not hot) coconut oil first.

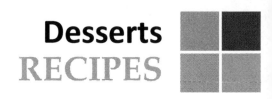

Place on plate with waxed paper, chill thoroughly, and store in airtight container in the refrigerator or on counter if less than 70 degrees in home.

* Inspired by Three Stone Hearth

Chocolate (Avocado) Pudding
GFCF/ SCD/GAPS/ Paleo/LOD/FG, Egg-Free/Nut-Free

To make FG, prepare without honey.

Ingredients
2 avocadoes
1/3-½ cup unsweetened cocoa or carob powder
1 cup of sweetener (honey, maple syrup, dates)

Directions
Blend all ingredients in blender or food processor until mixture is a little light. Chill and serve.

Sunflower Butter Brownies
GFCF/ SCD/GAPS/LOD/FG, Nut-Free

To make FG, prepare without honey (try maple syrup).

This is more of a "medium" oxalate recipe than low oxalate.

Ingredients
1 cup sunflower butter
1/3-1/2 cup raw honey
½ teaspoon baking soda
1 egg
½ teaspoon salt

Directions
Mix all ingredients and bake at 350 degrees for 20-30 minutes.

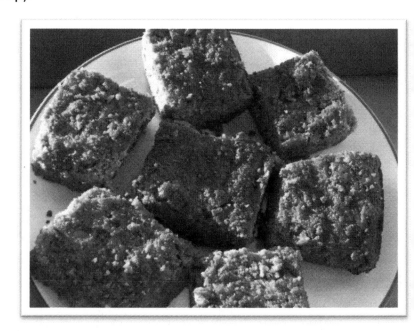

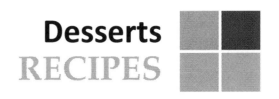

Chocolate Chip Cookies
GFCF/FG, Nut-Free

Ingredients
2 ¾ cups of GF flour blend
I use:
1 ½ cups sorghum flour
¾ cup potato starch (not potato flour)
½ cup tapioca starch (also known as tapioca flour)
½ teaspoon baking soda
2 teaspoons xanthan gum
½ teaspoon salt
¼ cup ghee
¼ cup coconut oil
½ cup cane sugar (evaporated cane sugar or white sugar)
½ cup brown sugar
2 teaspoons vanilla
2 eggs
1 bag of GFCF chips (I like Enjoy Life mini chips that are also soy-free)

Directions
Preheat over to 350 degrees.

Combine flour blend, baking soda, xanthan gum, and salt in a bowl and set aside. Cream ghee and coconut oil, then add cane sugar and brown sugar and blend together. Add eggs and vanilla and mix. Add flour blend, little by little, mixing into wet ingredients. Once thoroughly blended, add chips.

Form into balls, pressing down on them slightly. Place onto cookie sheet and bake in oven for 10-12 minutes or until lightly browned. Cool for a few minutes, then remove from cookie sheet and place on cooling rack.

Oat Flour Chocolate Chip Cookies
GFCF/FG, Nut-Free

If oats are tolerated, these cookies have virtually the exact flavor and texture of gluten-based chocolate chip cookies. Avoid nuts, for nut-free recipe.

Use certified gluten-free (GF) oats and oat flour. You can either grind all oats into the same flour texture, or blend some oat coarsely for a more "oatmeal" texture cookie.

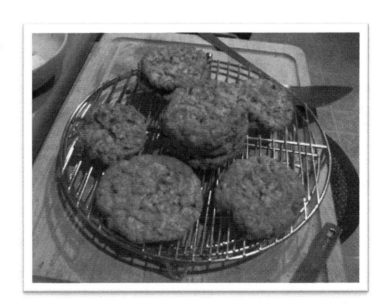

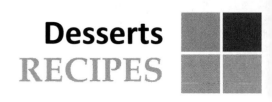

Ingredients

1 cup GF oat flour (you can also blend rolled oats into flour vs. using already milled flour)

1 ¼ cups rolled oats

½ teaspoon baking soda

½ teaspoon baking powder (GF and aluminum-free)

¼ teaspoon salt

¼ cup ghee

¼ cup coconut oil

½ cup cane sugar (evaporated cane sugar or white sugar)

½ cup brown sugar

1 egg

½ teaspoon vanilla

2 oz GFCF chocolate bar (grated)

¾ cup nuts (optional)

Directions

Preheat over to 375 degrees.

Measure rolled oats and blend in blender (Vitamix's grain grinder (pitcher) works great for this) into a fine or coarse flour. Combine oat flour and blended oats, baking soda, baking powder, and salt in a bowl and set aside.

Cream ghee and coconut oil, then add cane sugar and brown sugar and blend together. Add eggs and vanilla and mix.

Add flour blend, little by little, mixing into wet ingredients. Once thoroughly blended, add grated chocolate, chocolate chips, and nuts (optional).

Form into balls and place onto cookie sheet. Bake in oven for 10 minutes or until lightly browned. Cool for a few minutes, then remove from cookie sheet and place on cooling rack.

Chocolate Chip Almond Cookies
GFCF

Ingredients

1 cup GF oat flour

1 cup almond flour

¾ cup sugar (evaporated cane juice)

¼ cup date sugar or brown sugar

1 teaspoon xanthan gum

½ teaspoon baking soda

1 teaspoon salt

½ cup coconut/ghee mixed

1 egg

1 teaspoon gluten-free vanilla extract

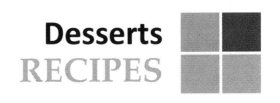

1 teaspoon almond extract
½ cup chocolate chips

Directions

Preheat oven to 350 degrees.

In a large mixing bowl, beat coconut/ghee with egg, brown sugar, granulated sugar, vanilla and almond extract. In separate bowl, combine dry ingredients.

Add flour mixture to wet ingredients, mixing thoroughly.

Stir in chocolate chips or nuts, if desired. Drop by tablespoons on baking sheet.

Bake at 350 degrees for 12-14 minutes.

Chocolate Bark
GFCF/Paleo, Nut-Free, Egg-Free

This is Paleo and Primal but not SCD/GAPS because of the chocolate. It's delicious and low in sugar. A square 1/12 of the recipe has only 1 gram of sugar plus whatever is in any dried fruit added. You can even make it sugar-free by using unsweetened chocolate and xylitol (corn-free). Can easily be made nut-free by avoiding adding nuts.

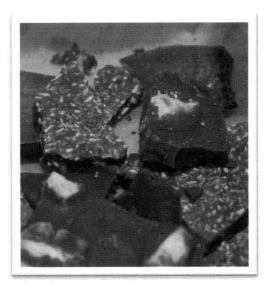

Ingredients

2 oz organic dark chocolate (dairy-free) bar, 65-75% cocoa
½ cup raw coconut oil
½ cup ghee, cocoa butter, or coconut oil
3 oz nuts, dried fruit, or trail mix
1-2 dried shredded coconut (no sulfur or sugar)

Directions

Melt dark chocolate in double boiler or in a pot on very low heat. Add coconut oil and ghee, stir on very low for 1-2 minutes, then remove from heat and finish melting the oils.

Line a small (6x8) Pyrex dish or baking sheet with parchment paper. Sprinkle the nuts, fruits and shredded coconut along the bottom of the dish. Pour the melted chocolate over the top and cover the nuts and fruit. Put in freezer, after 45minutes or so when it's hardening but not too frozen, cut the bark, then continue to freeze for 2 hours or until frozen.

Photo includes chocolate bark with shredded coconut and chunks of "No-Sugar" Coconut Bark.

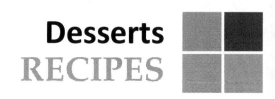
No-Sugar Coconut Bark
GFCF/SCD/GAPS/Paleo/LOD, Nut-Free, Egg-Free

Avoid almonds for LOD, and avoid almonds and almond extract for nut-free.

Ingredients
1.5 cup coconut butter
2 Tablespoons coconut oil
1 cup raw almonds (chopped) or other nut/seed
1 teaspoon vanilla extract
½ teaspoon Himalayan crystal salt

Optional ingredients
1/2 teaspoon almond extract
½ cup dried fruit like raisins, cranberries, currants or goji berries
1 cup unsweetened shredded coconut
2 Tablespoons xylitol

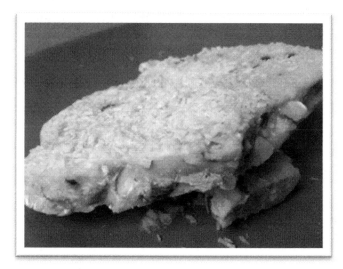

Directions
Line a 9x13 inch pan with parchment paper (along bottom and up sides). Toast almonds in pan (either with or without oil).

Melt coconut oil and coconut butter on double boiler, add vanilla extract, and salt.
Pour batter in pan and spread with a spatula. Sprinkle nuts, seeds or fruit throughout melted coconut butter and press into butter. Finally sprinkle shredded coconut onto the top.

Store in freezer or refrigerator. Serve cold.

Gelatin Hearts
GFCF/ Soy-free/ SCD/GAPS/Paleo/GAPS/Low oxalate, Nut-Free, Egg-Free

Gelatin Hearts are finger gelatin that you can pick up and eat with your fingers. It is two layers of gelatin with a strawberry heart in the middle.

Read instructions and get ingredients for everything ready. Start with the White Gelatin.

For gelatin, use a good quality gelatin from pasture-raised cows. If you are using gelatin packets, please note they are

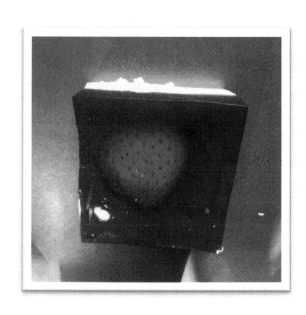

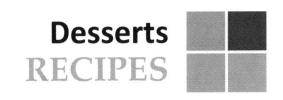

often 2 teaspoons rather than1 tablespoon so you will want to measure the amount. Delicious with no added sweetener. Use honey or no sweetener for SCD/GAPS.

White Gelatin Layer– Coconut Gelatin

Ingredients for White Gelatin
1 cup Water
1 cup coconut milk or cream
2 Tablespoons gelatin (use grass-fed type such as Bernard Jenson's), plus 1 teaspoon additional if you want them thicker.
1 Tablespoon honey or sweetener of your choice
¼ teaspoon Vanilla extrac*t*

Directions
White Coconut Layer: Put 1/2 <u>cold</u> water in a 1-quart bowl. Sprinkle gelatin on water and let it dissolve. Add 1/2 cup of <u>boiling</u> water – pour slowly, let sit, then stir well. Add coconut milk, honey and vanilla. Pour into bottom of flat-bottom pan 9 x 13 inches or two smaller pans (no greasing needed), and place in refrigerator to set.

Cut strawberries while white layer sets. Wash, de-stem, and cut strawberries in half. Cut a small V into the top of the strawberry to accentuate the heart shape if needed. Once white layer is set, place strawberry on top. Make Fruit Gelatin next. See assembly instructions for how to complete the layers.

Fruit Finger Gelatin
For the juice for this recipe, any type will work, fresh squeeze or bottled. A clear (not cloudy) juice is best in order to see the strawberry heart. Some good pink juices are homemade watermelon or strawberry juice). The juice used in the photo is black cherry.

Ingredients for Fruit Gelatin
1 cup of water
3 Tablespoons gelatin (plus one teaspoon if you want them on the firmer side)
2 cups juice

Directions for Fruit Gelatin
Put 1/2 <u>cold</u> water in a 1-quart bowl. Sprinkle gelatin on water and let it dissolve. Boil 1/2 cup of water, add 1 cup of fruit juice and heat until just about boiling – pour on top of gelatin slowly, let sit, then stir well. Add the second 1 cup of fruit juice and stir.

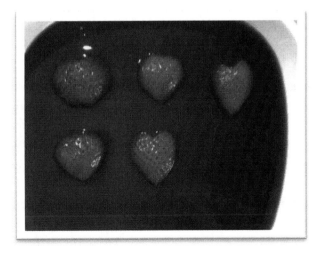

The sweetness of the gelatin depends on the juice. If your

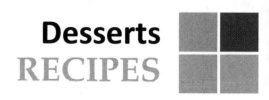

juice is more on the sour side, you may want to add a bit of sweetener of your choice – 1 Tablespoon should do the trick. If it's a sweeter juice but it tastes too "watered down," reduce the amount of boiling water and replace it with more fruit juice (that you heat along with the water).

Assembly Instructions
Pour on fruit gelatin covering about 1/3-1/2 of the strawberry. Let set in refrigerator 20 minutes. Note: if you pour it all at once, the strawberries will float and it will not work. Keep the extra liquid gelatin on the counter so it does not set. After about 20-30 pour remaining gelatin to cover strawberries and chill in refrigerator until done.

Gluten-Free Vanilla Cake & Cupcakes
GFCF/LOD/FG, Nut-free

The cupcakes are gluten-free and casein-free (GFCF) from a recipe I created through months of trial and food chemistry study (when to use baking powder vs. baking soda), etc. I'm quite pleased with the results – the cake is fluffy and no one even knew it was gluten-free – I got a "wow" when I mentioned it.

Gluten-Free Vanilla Cake
2 cups rice flour (white or brown)
2/3 cup potato starch
1/3 cup tapioca starch
1 ½ cups granulated sugar
1 Tablespoon GF baking powder
1 teaspoon baking soda
1 teaspoon salt
1 ½ teaspoons xanthan gum
1 cup coconut oil (flavorless, expeller-pressed)
4 eggs, room temperature
1 Tablespoon vanilla extract (gluten-free)
1 ½ cups milk (dairy or non-dairy – preferably unsweetened)

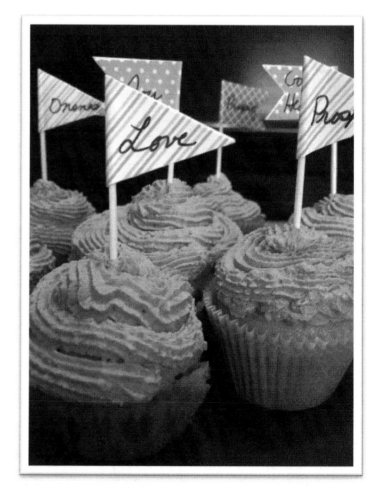

Instructions
Preheat the oven to 350 degrees. Batter makes enough for two 8 or 9-inch rounds or 24 cupcakes or 48 mini cupcakes. Grease and flour pans or get muffin tins and cupcake liners ready.
Place all dry ingredients in bowl starting with the sugar, then sifting in the flours and baking powder, baking soda, and xanthan gum.

Gently melt coconut oil in pan barely hot enough to melt. As the oil cools slightly (just enough not to "cook the eggs" when combined), in separate bowl combine the eggs and vanilla, then add the coconut oil.

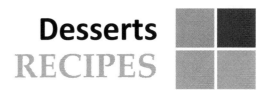

Once ready to combine everything, work swiftly at this point (attempting to have everything in the oven in 10 minutes). Alternate back and forth on the milk and flour by first adding half of the milk to the liquids and mix. Then add half the flour mix and blend. Add the final half of the milk while blending, then the remaining flour. The batter is a little thicker than gluten-containing cake mixes that most people are familiar with.

Bake mini cupcakes about 14-17 minutes, regular cupcakes a little longer, and cake pans will take about 30-35 minutes to back. Check them early to make sure they do not over cook. They are done, when a toothpick comes out clean. Once out of the oven, wait 10 minutes and then remove cake/cupcakes from pans and place on a baking rack to cool.

Coconut Whipped Cream Frosting
GFCF/SCD/GAPS/Paleo/LOD/FG

Use the **Coconut Whipped Cream** Recipe in "Milks and Butters" section. Spread on cake or cupcakes.

Chocolate Whipped Cream Frosting
GFCF/GAPS

This recipe can be made GAPS compliant by using honey instead of sugar. SCD doesn't allow cocoa.

This recipe can be made dairy-free using coconut cream that you can either buy from Wilderness Family Naturals or make buy using only the thick cream from a couple cans of coconut milk (not the watery liquid).

Directions
1 cup of coconut cream (chilled)
4 tablespoons cocoa (non-alkali or Dutch processed)
2 Tablespoons of sweetener (honey or sweetener of your choice)

Instructions
If you are using canned coconut milk, chill the cans for 30 minutes. Then open the cans and scoop solid/thick part of coconut into a bowl (use liquid in a smoothie or beverage).

Add the cocoa and sugar with a small amount of coconut cream and mix into a paste.

Once all the powder is incorporated, add all the rest of the coconut cream and beat with electric whisk or mixer, until whipped into peaks. If you desire more firm peaks, place bowl of cream in refrigerator again for 20-30 minutes. Then whip until finished.

Spread onto cake, or pipe onto cupcakes

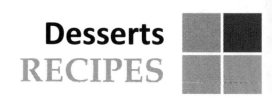
Intention Cupcakes

To make the "Intention Cupcakes" shown in the photo, either use these cupcake flags from Chronicle Books or create some of your own with paper and toothpicks, then write messages in permanent pen.

In the photo, all of the cupcake liners are from the "Pretty Cupcake Kit" except the hearts (which I believe are from Wilton), and are the minis. I love the cupcake liners from Chronicle Books, the regular-size has straighter sides that make them fit perfectly in to the muffin tins without crushing inward like many of the thin-papered and wide ones do.

Raw Dehydrated Macaroons
GFCF/SCD/GAPS/Paleo/LOD

To make SCD/GAPS use honey in place of maple – however, realize that the texture will be stickier. Technically maple is not a "raw" food, however the texture is best with maple. For LOD, Use low oxalate seed flour in place of almond flour.

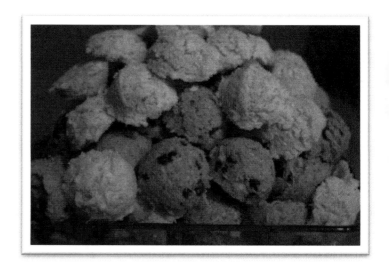

2 cups dried unsweetened coconut, finely shredded
½ cup almond flour, or other nut/seed flour (i.e. ground nuts/seeds)
¼ cup coconut butter
1/3 cup maple syrup (maple is not a raw food)
1 teaspoon vanilla extract
¼ teaspoon unrefined salt

Measure out dry ingredients. Place coconut butter jar in a bowl of warm/hot water to soften so coconut butter will scoop out more easily. Combine all wet ingredient into dry ingredients and mix thoroughly (with hands or a spoon). Scoop with a mini ice cream scoop (or about 1 -1 1/4 tablespoons or smaller if you prefer) and form into ball.

Place balls on dehydrator tray. Dehydrate at 130 degrees for the first hour, then turn down to 115 degrees for about 12-15 hours.

Cinnamon Almond Macaroons
GFCF/SCD/GAPS/LOD

Add to base macaroon mix:
1 teaspoon almond extract
1 teaspoon ground cinnamon
½ teaspoon ground cardamom

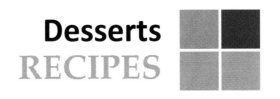

Use same instructions to finish recipe.

Chocolate Chip Macaroons
GFCF

Mini chocolate chips, dairy-free and soy-free such as Enjoy Life Foods

Add around 1/3 cup chocolate chips to the Macaroon dough. Follow Raw Dehydrated Macaroons recipe.

Pineapple Coconut Macaroons
GFCF/SCD/GAPS/LOD

2 ½ cups dried unsweetened coconut, finely shredded
¾ cups coconut butter
1 cup pineapple, chunks
1 cup of pineapple juice (from pineapple)

Blend pineapple in food processor until smooth.

Simmer pineapple juice down to 1 Tablespoon of "syrup" – this will take 5-10 minutes – watch it closely, at the end it will burn quickly if you are not careful.

Combine all ingredients in a bowl and mix with hands until thoroughly combined. Scoop with mini ice cream scoop or spoon and form into balls. Place balls on dehydrator tray.

Dehydrate at 115 degrees for about 12-24 hours.

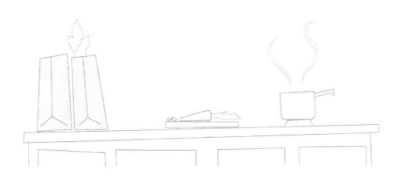

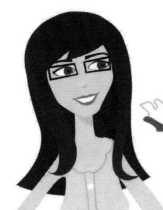

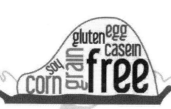

Fermented Foods

Probiotics

Non-Dairy Fermented Beverages
Kombucha • Coconut Kefir •
"Sodas"

Non-Dairy Fermented Foods
Raw sauerkraut • Fermented
sweet potato • Almond Yogurt

Dairy/Fermented Dairy
Raw Dairy • A1 and A2 Dairy
Yogurt • Wheys

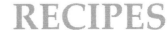

Fermented Foods Containing Good Bacteria

Yogurt and kefir: Yogurt and kefir, made from dairy, are excellent sources of good bacteria. Kefir is similar to yogurt but is easier to pour (homemade yogurt is thinner than store bought because it does not have extra milk solids or thickeners). Additionally, kefir (like kombucha) has good yeast to kill candida.

Young coconut kefir/kefired soda: Great alternatives for those who can't tolerate dairy. You get the benefit of the kefir cultures without the casein. The benefit to kefir is that it is a culture of bacteria and yeast. This culture kills yeast and is helpful for yeast overgrowth. The taste of young coconut kefir is pretty good and many kids like it and will drink it. Unfortunately, this drink is not made commercially and has to be made by hand. I have to admit it is a bit time consuming and touchy to make. The other thing to be aware of is that some people have sensitivity to coconut. Kefired soda is a similar sweet/sour, fizzy beverage that kids enjoy.

Lacto-fermented vegetables and fruits: Raw sauerkraut, cultured vegetables, and kim chi are types of cultured or fermented vegetables. All cultured foods are sour, a product of the acidic bacteria. You can really experience this with raw sauerkraut. It is very sour. While it took me a while to fully enjoy it, it grows on you and the sour flavor becomes very enjoyable. Some children love sauerkraut and its sour taste; others (especially those that don't like vegetables) will not touch it or need some time to get used to it. Fermented fruit is a wonderful option for children that do not like cultured vegetables.

Kombucha, a cultured food we don't hear too much about, but it is catching on very quickly. It is my favorite of the cultured foods. It is delicious and kids love it! Kombucha is often misclassified as "mushroom tea" leading people to believe it is some sort of mushroom boiled and made into a tea. This is not the case. It is a brew of sweetened black or green tea that is fermented with a culture of bacteria and yeast. The bacteria and yeast feed on the sugar and convert it into beneficial components that help with digestion, detoxification, immune function, cellular metabolism, etc. It is also used to treat constipation, candida, digestive disturbances, immune system problems like AIDS, cancer, headaches, and a variety of heart-supportive treatments.

Whey contains a great deal of minerals. It is also a wonderful source of lactobacillus bacteria. One tablespoon of whey with some water will help digestion. Whey added to vegetable broths assists in the assimilation of potassium and other minerals. Breast milk is higher in whey than other animal milks and an important addition to infant formula.

Whey is often used in the fermentation of vegetables and fruits. Vegetable fermentation can be made with or without whey, but fruit ferments must include whey for proper fermentation. Whey assists in the fermentation of grains and beans by breaking down phytic acid, which blocks absorption of calcium, magnesium, copper, iron and zinc. Soaking (in a liquid mixture of water and whey) also neutralizes enzyme inhibitors, increasing enzyme activity and digestibility

Non-Dairy Fermented Beverages

Kombucha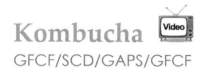
GFCF/SCD/GAPS/GFCF

For SCD/Gaps, use honey in place of sugar

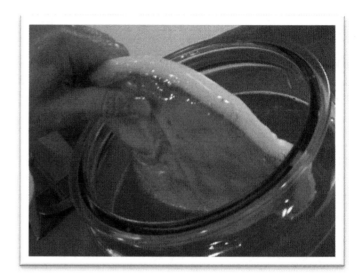

Ingredients
1 gallon water
1 cup sugar (plain white is always recommended in recipes but I use evaporated cane juice)
4 Tablespoons black or green tea (herbal will not work)
2 cups kombucha drink from already made batch or amount used to store Kombucha culture

Directions
Mix water and sugar and bring to a boil in a pot.
Turn off heat and add tea. Cover and steep 15 minutes
Strain tea into glass or ceramic (crock) container. Something wide, preferably as wide as or wider than it is tall. Allow to cool to room temperature.

Add the 2 cups mature kombucha liquid and place the kombucha culture in the liquid with the firm opaque (whiter) side up.

Cover with cloth and store in a warm place (ideally 70-85 degrees). If it's cooler it will work but will take longer to fully brew.

After a few days to 1 week you will notice a skin forming on the surface. It can take anywhere from 7-28 days depending on the temperature and size of your batch. Taste the liquid by inserting a straw. It's done right when it's between sweet and sour/vinegar taste and is fizzy. If you let it go too long it will taste too vinegary. Once it reaches the acidity you like, start a new batch and store your mature kombucha in the refrigerator. You now have two mothers, the original one you started with and the new one (the skin that formed on your first batch). Use either the new or the old mother in your new batch and pass the other to a friend or compost it.

Young Coconut Kefir
GFCF/BED/Not officially SCD/GAPS/Paleo/FG

Young coconut water has complex sugars that are not allowed on SCD. However, my suspicion is that the fermentation process may break down the sugars into monosaccharides.

First, remove the 1-1/2 to 2 cups of water inside the young coconut and use it to make kefir. To do this, lay the coconut on its side and shave several layers off the bottom until a circle appears. If you keep on shaving, two more circles will appear and you'll have what looks like a face with two eyes and a mouth. Place the young coconut in your kitchen drain so that the point fits into the drain. (This just holds the coconut steady.) Take a sharp object like a carrot peeler or apple corer and poke it through the bigger (mouth) hole. Carve out the hole, making it bigger, and then flip the coconut over onto a glass jar to let the water pour out.

Use the water from four coconuts with one package of starter, let it sit on the counter for 24-48 hours, and you're all set. You'll know it's done when the color changes to a milky white and there's a bit of bubbling or foam on top. This means all the sugar has been removed. When you drink it, make sure it tastes tart and tangy. This is another sign that all the sugar is gone.

You can also use water kefir grains or even dairy kefir grains.

Special Notes: You can use about 1/4 cup from your first batch to "transfer" the friendly bacteria to your next batch of kefir. Do this up to seven times with one package of starter. And when the weather turns cold, warm the liquid to about 90 degrees before adding the starter. Then place the glass jar into an insulated container so it will maintain a steady temperature of about 70 degrees while fermenting.

Hibiscus and Rose Hip Soda
GFCF/ SCD/GAPS/Paleo/Gaps/BED

This was originally made with agave nectar. Instead, I am using sugar (evaporated cane juice). You could try honey for SCD; however, it may not ferment as well because of honey's antimicrobial properties. You can try Lakanto for BED.

Makes 2 quarts

Ingredients
¼ cup dried hibiscus flowers (purchased from an herb store)
1 Tablespoon dried rose hips
½ cup evaporated cane juice
½ cup kefir grains, or 1 cup yogurt whey
½ organic lemon
Filtered water

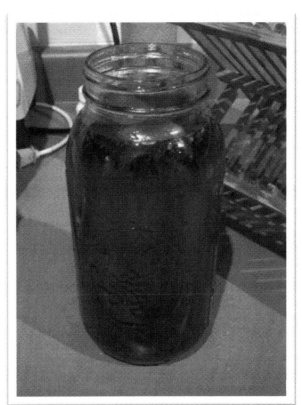

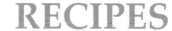

Directions

Put the hibiscus, rose hips, evaporated cane juice and whey or kefir grains in a 2-quart jar. Squeeze the juice from the lemon into the jar and add the rind as well. Pour in enough filtered water to fill the jar.

Screw the lid onto the jar and put it in a warm place for 2 days.

Strain into two glass bottles with screw tops. Put an even amount into both bottles. If they are 1-quart bottles, they should be full; if they are 1-liter bottles, add enough water to fill to the top. Screw the lids on tightly, label and date the bottles, and return to the warm place for another 2-3 days, or until the soda becomes slightly bubbly.

Transfer to the fridge. When you are ready to drink the soda, open the bottles carefully because they may have built up carbonation. Open them outside or over a sink. Turn the lid very slowly to see if the drink begins to release foam. If so, then allow it to release some of the carbon dioxide by not opening the bottle all the way and letting out some of the pressure, then opening it more and more, bit by bit. This way you won't lose your drink to its carbonation.

From "Full Moon Feast" by Jessica Prentice

Non- Dairy Fermented Foods

Nut Yogurt
GFCF/SCD/GAPS/Paleo/BED/FG

For FG, use any nut other than almonds. For LOD use coconut milk, pumpkinseed milk, or combination of LOD nuts/seeds.

Ingredients
1 1/3 cup whole, raw almonds, walnuts, hazelnuts and/or macadamias (soak 8-12 hours)
1-2 Tablespoons raw honey
3 cups water
Yogurt starter (GI ProStart by GI ProHealth or Klaire CulturAid Yogurt Starter)

Directions
Rinse nuts. Soak nuts for 8-12 hours. Drain and rinse nuts.

Put drained nuts into blender with 3 cups of fresh water.

Add 2 tablespoons of honey or a couple pitted dates and blend for 2-3 minutes.

Pour the nut milk through nut milk bag to separate the milk from nut meal.

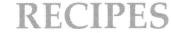

Heat nut milk to 160 degrees (This will keep the yogurt from separating). When it reaches 160 degrees, you can begin to cool it. Some people simmer nut milk when using cashews.

Cool nut milk to 105 degrees.

Add yogurt starter based on label's instructions. Typically it's about 1/8 teaspoon of yogurt starter to the milk, per quart of yogurt. Stir well with whisk.

Place container(s) in yogurt maker or in dehydrator at 95-105 degrees. Leave lids off individual yogurt containers during fermentation to avoid condensation on lids that may thin the finished yogurt. Ferment for 8 hours.

Place in the fridge overnight or at least for hours (overnight is better)

For thicker yogurt, strain the yogurt into a bowl lined with cheesecloth to remove liquid*. Drain for about an hour, or longer for thicker yogurt. By pressing the dripped yogurt further, you can make something that resembles cheese.

* Straining is optional. Homemade nut milk yogurt is thinner than commercial versions.

Nut Cream Cheese (Strained Yogurt)
GFCF/SCD/GAPS/Paleo/BED

Drip nut yogurt by placing a strainer/sieve in the top of a bowl.

Place a cloth in the strainer.

Pour the nut yogurt into the towel-lined strainer.

Cover the strainer with a plate or a cloth and leave it for 5-8 hours.

When it is done, you will have a nut cream cheese.

Vegetable and Fruit Kebabs with Nut Yogurt Dipping Sauce
GFCF/ SCD/GAPS/GAPS/Paleo

For FG, use complaint fruit (pear, mango, golden delicious apples, etc.)

Kids love things "on a stick," so fruit kebabs are a hit. For kids new to eating vegetables, the combination of foods they like (fruit) with unknown foods (vegetables) is a good way to encourage exploration of (and success in eating) vegetables.

Any fruits you like (mango, pear, berry, melon)
Vegetables that are good raw (red pepper, cherry tomato, jicama, celery, peas, cucumber, cooked and cooled butternut squash chunks.

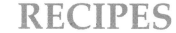

Condiments and Sauces
RECIPES

Ingredients

Dipping sauce
1 cup of nut milk yogurt
1 cup of fresh or frozen ORGANIC strawberries, peaches or other fruit
1-2 Tablespoons raw honey

Directions

Mash fruit with a fork or puree in a blender and add a splash of the milk yogurt (enough to get it to spin) and honey.

Place appropriately sized chucks of alternating fruits and vegetables on a bamboo skewer.

Serve sauce in a fun bowl.   Place skewer on plate with bowl of dipping sauce in the center.

Raw Sauerkraut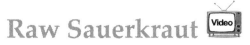
GFCF/ SCD/GAPS/Paleo/LOD/BED/FG

- Ceramic crock and a plate or other jar that fits inside crock to hold the cabbage down
- 1 quart or 2 liter jar filled with water (scrub the outside)
- Cloth cover such as muslin or kitchen towel

5 lbs/2 kilograms cabbage (Green or red/purple)
3 tablespoons/45 milliliters sea salt

1. Rinse cabbage. Retain two outer cabbage leaves. Grate cabbage by hand with mandolin or in food processor, finely or coarsely.
2. Place cabbage in bowl. Sprinkle salt on cabbage as you go. The salt pulls water out of cabbage and creates the brine so it can ferment and sour without rotting. The salt also keeps the cabbage crunchy by inhibiting organisms and enzymes that soften it.
3. You can add other vegetables such as carrots, ginger, radishes, onions, garlic, leafy greens, seaweed, beets, turnips and burdock roots. Juniper berries are common. For consistent results, I typically use a majority (75%) cabbage with some of these other vegetables for flavor and variety. You can try almost anything, but without a starter, vegetables containing natural lactobacillus are the best such as cabbage and root vegetables including beets, radishes, turnips, and carrots.
4. Mix ingredients and pack into crock. Pack a small amount into the crock a little at a time and tamp it down with your fist or a kitchen implement like a potato masher. You can also massage cabbage with your hands, and then tamp down. The goal is to force water out of cabbage, pack the kraut tightly, and press out any air. If you'd like, you can place a cabbage heart (the center of the cabbage) in the center of the sauerkraut in the crock. The center pickles and leaves you with very crispy, crunchy cabbage that you can eat with your fingers—this is often fun for children.

Condiments and Sauces
RECIPES

5. Place cabbage leaves in crock on top of packed cabbage to keep any shredded cabbage from floating to the surface of the water. Place the plate over the leaves to keep everything down. Add a weighted jar (filled with water works) to top to act as a weight. The goal is to keep EVERYTHING (except the jar) under water. The water is formed by the liquid in the cabbage and the salt. Let it sit for 6 hours or so and see if the water line rises above the cabbage. If there is not an inch and a half of water, add salt water in the ratio of 1 tablespoon salt to 1 cup of water. Salt inhibits mold growth, but too much salt slows good bacteria. As such, you want to be fairly accurate with your salt/cabbage and salt water proportions.

6. Cover with fabric cloth and tie with a string or large rubber band. Make sure it goes all the way around so no bugs can get it.
   a. If you use a Harsch crock, the process (in steps 5 and 6) is simple. Instead of needing a plate and weight, specially made weights are included. Place the plates on top of the cabbage making sure the water is over the top of the vegetables. Place lid on top and fill rim with water to form water seal. No fabric is necessary.

7. Ferment for 2-8 weeks or more. Personally, I like long ferments of 8 weeks or more. Because my home (in San Francisco) is very cool all year round (resembling a cellar), the kraut turns out great every time. Always sour and crunchy. Never soft.
   The types and amounts of bacteria differ in the raw sauerkraut as the fermentation changes over time. For this reason, I like Sandor Katz's suggestion of "eating it as you go." Make a large batch. After two weeks, "harvest" one jar or one week's worth. Pack the sauerkraut back up and set aside to ferment. After that jar is finished, harvest another jar in the next week. Continue for eight to ten weeks or whenever it is done. This ensures that you get the various bacteria types and counts over time.

Additional notes:
- If you live in a warm climate, you will want to invest in a Harsch crock. They help insulate the sauerkraut with its thick ceramic. The crock keeps the kraut from getting mushy in hot weather. The weighted "plate" inside with an air tight water sealed lid keeps air out but allows gasses to escape.
- You can make sauerkraut with whey but it is not necessary and I've never noticed any difference either way. More importantly, whey is from yogurt and contains casein—something many people are trying to avoid with sauerkraut. You can also use a cultured vegetable starter such as the one Donna Gates has on BodyEcology.com. I like to do things the "old fashioned way" without a starter—it feels empowering.
- There is another method seen in books and online. This method typically doesn't weight the sauerkraut down, they use a starter, an airtight lid, and only ferment them 3-7 days. Be aware not to use this method for long ferments; otherwise, you will blow the top of your ferment.

Variation and note on salt: You can use half the salt by substituting seeds (an even mix of celery, caraway, and dill). Although, the original recipe uses only salt, it is not "salty" in taste—especially the longer it ferments.

*I adapted this recipe from Sandor Katz's sauerkraut recipe and his book, **Wild Fermentation**. This is one of my favorite books on fermenting everything. And he has a new book, *The Art of Fermentation*.

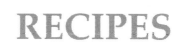

Apple Kraut
GFCF/ SCD/GAPS/LOD/BED/FG

This is the most kid-friendly way to eat raw sauerkraut. Use green apples for BED. To make FG, use pear instead of apple.

Ingredients
Raw sauerkraut
Apples

Directions
Grate apple (peeled or unpeeled). Mix equal parts kraut and apple. Enjoy!

Variation: You can grate carrots into the mix. You can also make a variation with applesauce instead of grated apple. Place applesauce and sauerkraut into food processor and puree.

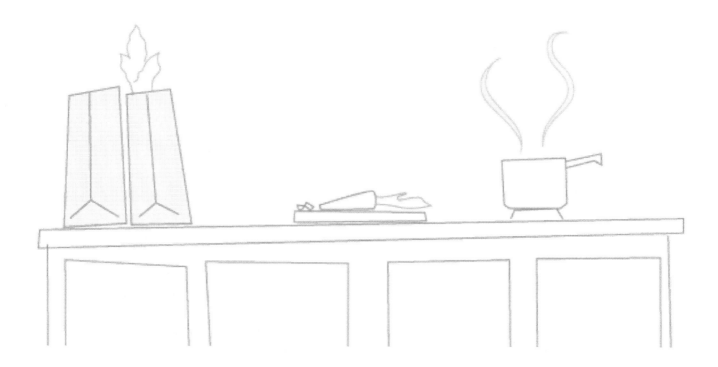

Dairy / Fermented Dairy

Raw Dairy

Dairy causes a great deal of controversy among nutrition consultants. Some say dairy products are vitally important, others suggest using only non-fat and low fat products, while others say the decrease in lactase enzyme in adults is evidence that we are not supposed to consume milk products past early childhood. Vegans say that cow milk is for cows, and absolutely not for humans.

There is some truth and some falsehood to each of these notions. However, we rarely dispute the most important fact– that milk should be consumed raw – as nature intended.

Dairy is one of the most common food sensitivities and allergies. New researchers and clinicians such as Dr. Mercola (www.mercola.com) believe that the problems with dairy stem from pasteurization, as this process:

Kills the natural enzymes
Kills good bacteria (that fights bad bacteria)
Reduces vitamin content and destroys vitamins C, B12 and B6
Alters the molecular structure of the protein molecules possibly causing casein intolerance
Promotes pathogens and is associated with allergies
Contributes to increases in tooth decay, colic in infants, growth problems in children, osteoporosis, arthritis, heart disease and cancer.

Calves fed pasteurized milk don't thrive and often die before adulthood. The homogenization process that emulsifies the fat into the milk so it doesn't separate is also harmful, especially to the heart – increases the rates of heart disease. Ultra-pasteurization is even worse than standard pasteurization methods, used to get rid of heat-resistant bacteria and give it a longer shelf life; this process takes milk from a chilled temperature to above the boiling point in less than two seconds.

Safety

Public health officials warn that raw milk poses the risk of transmitting bacteria such as listeria, E. coli and salmonella. Pasteurization was instituted in the 1920s to combat tuberculosis, infant diarrhea, fever and other diseases caused by poor animal nutrition and dirty production methods of mass produced milk. Pasteurization kills these bacteria while extending the milk's shelf life - the dairy industry profits while consumers and cows suffer. With organically raised cows, stainless steel tanks and milking machines, refrigerated trucks and inspection methods allow pasteurization to be eliminated.

The biggest public campaign against raw milk has been centered on the fear about safety, so let's examine this much more closely. The Weston A. Price Foundation web site (http://westonaprice.org) states:

Condiments and Sauces
RECIPES

"Except for a brief hiatus in 1990, raw milk has always been for sale commercially in California, usually in health food stores, although I can remember a period when it was even sold in grocery stores. Millions of people consumed commercial raw milk during that period and although the health department kept an eagle eye open for any possible evidence of harm, not a single incidence was reported. During the same period, there were many instances of contamination in pasteurized milk, some of which resulted in death."

While it is certainly possible to become sick from drinking contaminated raw milk, it is also possible to become sick from almost any food source. Because of the great care taken to produce raw milk safely, there is rarely a problem with contamination from raw milk. However, because of potential health concerns *if* the milk is contaminated, pregnant women and the immune compromised should only consume raw milk after they feel comfortable with their own analysis of the facts.

Commercial vs. Raw vs. Organic

Much of vegans concern over milk is regarding how poorly the cows are treated. There is nothing natural about how commercial dairy cows used to produce milk are raised - selectively bred to generate the most milk, fed a diet high in protein, kept in confined spaces, and fed antibiotics to combat poor living conditions, treatment, and disease — these cows are not naturally raised healthy animals. They pump out three to four times the amount of milk compared to their free-range counterparts and die prematurely.

Cows raised for raw milk production are often old-fashioned Jersey and Guernsey cows. Because they are well cared for, there is no need to add large quantities of antibiotics to their "feed." In fact, in many cases these cows are not fed feed. They graze on large acreages of pesticide-free green grass and get plenty of sunlight. This creates an abundant amount of vitamins A & D that is present in the butterfat.

Be aware that some cows that are raised for organic (but pasteurized) milk are often not raised on their natural diet of green grass and are fed corn or barley based feeds. While organic is certainly superior to commercial milk, it is lacking many of the properties of raw milk due to pasteurization (and often homogenization).

Whole Fat Milk

The low-fat and non-fat milk recommendations of many nutritionists of the past did not take into consideration the importance of the essential milk fatty acids and fat soluble vitamins. Even today, most people think they are doing a good thing by consuming low fat milk. When we are talking about pasteurized milk products deficient in all of the important qualities of pasture-raised, raw dairy - good essential fatty acids, vitamins A & D, enzymes, probiotics, and more — this may be true.

Vitamins A and D are needed for proper assimilation of calcium and protein. The fat in milk is rich in fatty acids, which protect against disease and stimulate the immune system. It contains glyco-spingolipids, which prevent intestinal distress, and conjugated linoleic acid that has strong anti-cancer properties and aids fat burning.

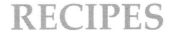

Additionally, low-fat milk has powdered skim milk added, and in the process of powdering it, the cholesterol is dangerously oxidized – creating a substance that is damaging to the arteries. It is not the fat in milk, but the oxidation of the cholesterol added to milk that creates heart disease. This high heat drying process also creates cross-linked proteins and nitrate compounds, which are carcinogenic. Additionally, free glutamic acid is created which is toxic to the nervous system and a big problem for many with autism - one of the many reasons milk is not tolerated by children with autistic spectrum disorders.

Digestibility

The natural enzymes, probiotics, and unadulterated proteins make raw milk much easier to digest and assimilate than commercial milk products. The process of heating the milk during pasteurization alters the protein and is believed to be one of the factors creating the high rates of casein sensitivity.

Milk and cheeses from raw milk contain a full array of enzymes and are more easily digested. When cheese is eaten unheated it is even more digestible. In addition, when milk is fermented, casein is predigested, making digestion of casein easier.

While it is true that some populations do not continue to produce lactase, (the enzyme to break down lactose and prevent lactose-intolerance) additional decline in lactase in adults is due to overuse of antibiotics and the deficiency in good bacteria that results. Raw milk and lactobacillus in fermented milk have adequate amounts of enzymes present to break down the milk for easy digestion, while pasteurization kills these enzymes and probiotics.

Research and Resources

Because of this fear that has been created about unpasteurized dairy, most states don't even sell raw dairy—California, Connecticut, Montana and New Mexico do. If your state does not sell raw milk commercially, you can often get it from the farm, a co-op, cow share or other non-commercial means.

As this is such an important decision, especially for children and the immune compromise, it is essential for you to do your own research to feel personally comfortable before proceeding with adding raw milk to your diet. Here are a couple resources below:

- RealMilk.com
- OrganicPastures.com

A1 and A2 Dairy

We often think of casein – all casein– as the enemy with milk. There are actually many forms of casein including alpha, beta and kappa casein. Scientists and farmers in New Zealand have been studying the effects of two types of beta casein—A1 vs. A2 beta-casein—and have found that A1 beta-casein is the protein in most

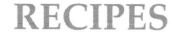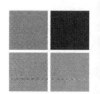

(Holstein) dairy cows. Goats, sheep and buffalo, as well as certain dairy cows (Jersey and Guernsey) produce primarily A2 beta casein.

The variance between A1 and A2 beta casein is a different amino acid at position 67—Histidine for A1 milk vs. Proline for A2. This small change causes A1 milk to be broken down during digestion into an opiate compound, BMC-7 (beta casomorphin 7); whereas, A2 does not.

There are a few studies suggesting that the A1 beta-casein molecule and the resulting BMC-7 opiate may be responsible for many, if not all problems, with the casein in milk – increased risk of heart disease, type I diabetes, autism, and schizophrenia.

One of the reasons raw milk may not cause negative casein reactions may be because raw milk dairy farms often have higher numbers of cows such as Guernsey and Jersey cows that produce much lower levels of A1 milk. It is also postulated that pasteurization or processing (cheese making) may also have an effect on the level of opiates in the milk.

Goat, sheep, buffalo produce primarily A2 milk. Some people may choose to try different types of milk and see if any work better for them. See article on A1 & A2 dairy at NourishingHope.com

Fermented Dairy

Yogurt
GF (not CF)/ SCD/GAPS/LOD/FG

Makes 1 quart

Ingredients
1 quart pasteurized whole milk, non-homogenized
1/8 teaspoon yogurt start 1/2 cup good quality commercial plain yogurt, or 1/2 cup yogurt from previous batch
Candy thermometer

Directions
Yogurt is easy to make—neither a yogurt-maker nor a special culture is necessary. The final product may be thinner in consistency than commercial yogurt.

Gently heat the milk to 180 degrees and allow to cool to about 110 degrees. Stir in yogurt and place in a shallow glass, enamel or stainless steel container. Cover the container and place in a warm oven at about 150 degrees or a gas oven with a pilot light overnight. In the morning transfer to the refrigerator. Throughout the day, use paper towels to absorb excess whey that is created during the yogurt making process.

Variation: Raw Milk Yogurt
GF (not CF)/ SCD/GAPS/BED

Ingredients
1 quart raw milk
1/8 teaspoon yogurt starter or ¼ cup yogurt from last batch (GI Pro Health makes a yogurt starter)

Directions
Warm milk on stove to 105 degrees; be careful not to go above. Put a couple ounces of warm milk into a small bowl or jar and add the starter or yogurt and stir well, blending it with a spoon. Pour warm milk into quart sized container, along with yogurt starter.

Place a kitchen towel or cloth over jar and secure with a rubber band.

Remove trays from dehydrator and jar at the bottom of the dehydrator. Set heat between 95-100 degrees, 105 degrees is a bit warm for raw milk but does activate some of the yogurt bacteria better. Heat in dehydrator for 24 hours. Once done, refrigerate.

Whey/Cream Cheese
GF (not CF)/ SCD/GAPS/BED

Yogurt can be separated into whey and curds (cream cheese). The cream cheese will have live lactobacillus acidophilus in it, making it a far healthier alternative to store bought cream cheese.

Pour yogurt into a large strainer covered with a muslin cloth or kitchen towel over a bowl. Leave on the counter at room temperature as the whey (a clear yellowish liquid) drains into the bowl below. After a few hours, tie up the towel with yogurt inside around a wooden spoon and place spoon on top of a taller container so more whey can drip out. The full process typically takes 1-2 days. Once complete, store whey in a jar with lid in the refrigerator. Cream cheese will keep for about a month and the whey will keep for 3-4 months or longer.

Dairy Kefir
GF (not CF)/LOD/BED/FG

1 quart milk (pasteurized, goat, raw)
1 tablespoon kefir grains

Pour milk into jar (leaving several inches of space or 1/3 of jar). Add kefir grains and screw lid on. Place on counter at room temperature for 24-48 hours. Gentle shake jar every so often.

Strain grains. Use spoon to separate grains and stir kefir through strainer. Kefir will separate and become effervescent the longer it's fermented.

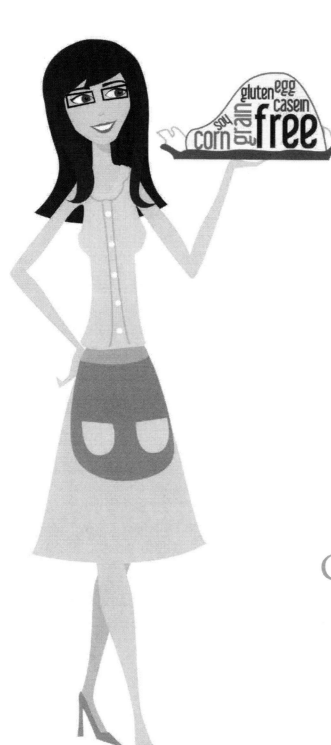

Condiments and
Sauces

Honey-Mustard Dipping Sauce
GFCF/SCD/GAPS/Paelo/Egg-Free/Nut-Free

Ingredients
½ cup raw honey
½ cup Dijon (or other GF) mustard

Directions
Mix and serve as a dipping sauce for chicken nuggets, meatballs, or as a dressing for salads (dilute with water and/or apple cider vinegar if desired).

BBQ Dipping Sauce
GFCF, Egg-Free/Nut-Free

To ensure soy-free, choose a soy-free Worchestershire sauce, leave out the Worchestershire sauce, or use the soy-free recipe at See www.tacanow.org.

Ingredients
1 cup organic ketchup
1 1/2 tablespoons raw apple cider vinegar
2 tablespoons raw honey
¼ teaspoon onion powder
1/8 teaspoon garlic powder
1/8 teaspoon salt and black pepper
1 teaspoon Worchestershire sauce (most contain SOY) (optional)

Blend all of the above until smooth. Serve as a dipping sauce for chicken nuggets, meatballs, and other foods.

GFCF Ranch Dressing Dip
GFCF, Egg-Free/Nut-Free

Can be made nut-free with hemp cream in place of cashew cream. Can even be made egg-free using an egg-free mayo.

Ingredients
3/4 cup cashew cream or non-dairy yogurt
1/2 cup mayonnaise
1 teaspoon of lemon juice or apple cider vinegar (with yogurt, less lemon or vinegar may be needed, add to taste)
1 teaspoon parsley (dried)
3/4 teaspoon dill
1/4 teaspoon garlic
¼ teaspoon onion
1/8 teaspoon salt

Condiments and Sauces
RECIPES

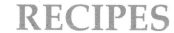

DIrections

Blend 1/2 cup cashews plus 1/2 cup hot or boiling water in blender until a thick cream.

Add rest of ingredients and whisk until blended together.

Chill and serve as a dip. Can be thinned with a non-dairy milk and used as a Ranch salad dressing.

Inspired by Sueson Vess.

No-Mato (Tomato-Free) Sauce
GFCF/ SCD/Gaps/Paleo, Egg-Free

Ingredients
5-6 carrots, chopped
1 red/purple beet, peeled and chopped
1 small or 1/2 large onion, peeled and chopped
2 celery stalks, chopped
1 ½ cups water

Directions
Place all chopped and prepared vegetables and water into a pot. Once water boils, reduce heat, cover and simmer for 50-60 minutes. Vegetables should be soft when pierced. Then place an emersion blender in pot and blend until smooth (or place contents in blender and puree). Use in place of tomato sauce as desired.

Place chips in oven to bake for 15-20 minutes. Depends on the oven and temperature. It's better to go lower and slower. If leaves are brown, they taste burnt—you want them mostly green. Between 325-350 degrees is good.

You can also make these in the dehydrator.

Indian "Yogurt" Sauce with Greens
GFCF/ SCD/Gaps, Egg-Free

If you use cashew cream, add extra lime juice.

Ingredients

1 cup of yogurt (non-dairy, or homemade dairy yogurt if tolerated) or cashew cream
½ inch of fresh peeled ginger
2 scallions
½ green chile pepper
1/3 cup green herbs or leafy greens (cilantro, parsley, basil, mint, and/or kale – a combination with some herbs and greens is often good)
Juice of 1 lime or lemon juice (I prefer lime)

1 ½ teaspoon salt

Directions
Blend all of the herbs and spices together in the food processor. Add the lime juice and a couple tablespoons of yogurt (or cream) process further. Add the salt to taste. Swirl the green sauce lightly into the yogurt or mix thoroughly depending on desired appearance and taste.

Great topping for Chickpea Flour Pancakes.

Cranberry Apple Pear Sauce
GFCF/SCD/GAPS/Paleo, Egg-Free, Nut-Free

Ingredients
3 apples, peeled, cored and chopped
3 pears, peeled, cored and chopped
1 package of frozen or fresh cranberries (12 oz)

Splash of orange juice (1-2 oz)
½-1 Tablespoon maple syrup (or honey on SCD/GAPS)

Directions
Place apples, pears, cranberries, and orange juice in pot. Turn heat to low and simmer for 25 minutes. Once cranberries have popped and sauce is cooked down, add maple syrup to taste. My preference is a sweet-sour blend, not too sweet, just enough maple to take away the strong tart flavor—the amount of sweetener will depend on the type of apples you use, and how you like it.

Pear Sauce or Apple Sauce
GFCF/ SCD/GAPS/FG/FS, Egg-Free/Nut-Free

Make Feingold and Failsafe by using peeled pears, or peeled golden delicious apples.

Ingredients
6-12 pears or apples (make as little or as much as you'd like)
Water

Directions
If salicylates are of concern, you'll want to peel the fruit before cooking.

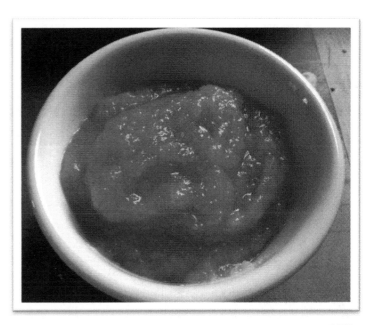

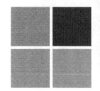
Wash pears or apples. If salicylates are not of concern, and you have a food mill (you do not need to peel them.

Chop fruit into quarters and place in large pot. Add about 1 inch of water to the bottom of the pot. Simmer on low for about 25 minutes. Stir a few times.

Fruit will cook down into sauce. If seeds, stems or skins are still on fruit, scoop fruit into food mill and turn the crank over a bowl. Skins will separate, and fruit sauce will fall into bowl.

Pear sauce is ready to serve.   If child likes it very smooth like baby food, blend one more time through food processor.

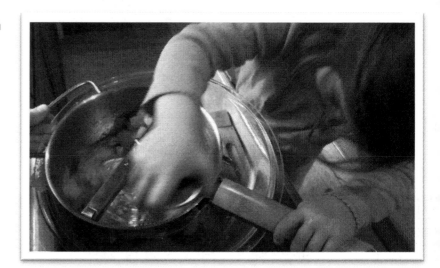

White Bean Hummus
GFCF/ SCD/GAPS/FG/FS, Egg-Free/Nut-Free

Make FS by eliminating the sesame tahini, and use sunflower oil instead of olive oil.

Ingredients
1 cup dry white beans (soak for 8-12 hours and rinse well and cook for 45 minutes until soft)
2 tablespoons olive oil
2 tablespoons lemon juice (or the juice of one lemon)
1-2 teaspoons finely minced garlic
1/4 cup sesame tahini (optional, eliminate if not on SCD for 3 months)
1 teaspoon salt

Directions
Combine in a food processor and mix well.

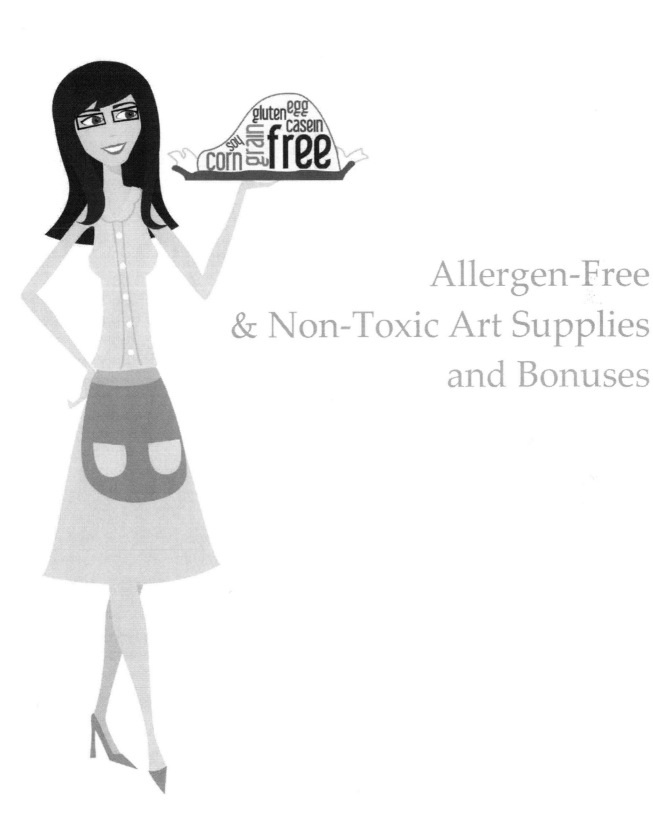

Allergen-Free
& Non-Toxic Art Supplies
and Bonuses

Gluten-Free Playdough
GFCF

Playdough is a fun and creative art medium. However, for gluten-free kids, Play-doh is not an option, as Play-doh brand contains gluten. Since gluten can absorb through the skin and (if your kids are like mine) kids often eat playdough, gluten-free playdough is the solution!

I have made many batches of playdough – some a total failure – so I'm here to share my learning and the recipe that works every time.

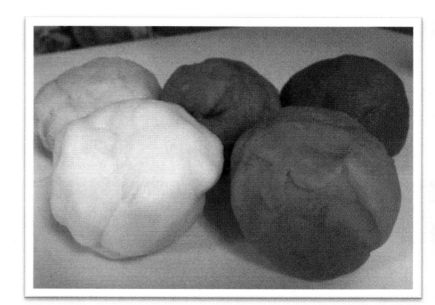

Ingredients
3/4 Cup White Rice Flour
3/4 Cup Cornstarch
3/4 Cup Salt
1 Tablespoon Cream of Tartar (same thing as tartaric acid powder – NOT tartar sauce)
2 teaspoons olive or seed oil
1 ½ Cup Water, hot but not boiling
Natural food coloring, as desired

Directions
Add all dry ingredients in a pot. Add vegetable oil, then the water, and continue to mix until thoroughly combined. Then turn on heat. Heat the pot on the stove over low heat – stir continuously for about 3 minutes. When the dough pulls away from the sides into a big ball, place dough into glass bowl.

Once cool enough to handle. Divide into 3-5 pieces. Add several drops of natural food coloring to the ball and massage until you get the color you desire. I like to make an indentation in the ball, drop in the food coloring, fold the ball over so the color is in the middle, and slowly knead until color is blended. If the dough is too wet, add cornstarch. If it's too dry, massage in a bit of water.

I find that when I add coloring it gets a bit too wet and sticky. I usually let is dry out for a few hours here and there (maybe 2 or 3 hours a few times – too many hours and it will get crusty around the edges). Then it's the perfect texture and not sticky any more. While you can also knead a bit of cornstarch in each batch, if you have a bit of sensory sensitivity, (like I must), you may not like that – so I use my palms.

Store in an airtight container. I do not store mine in the refrigerator and it stays fresh for 6 months.

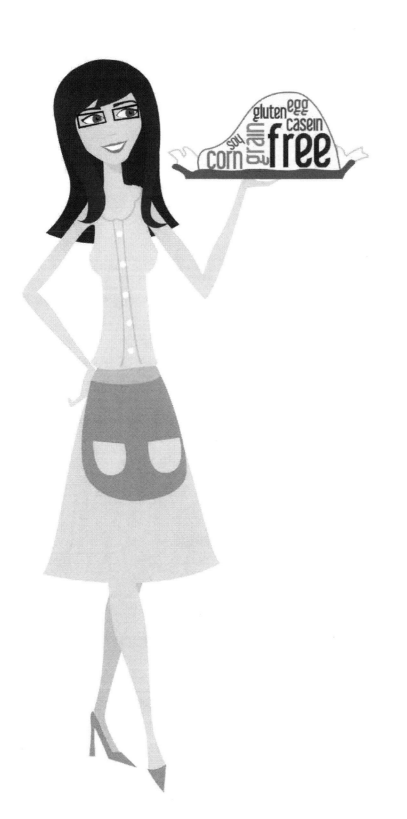

Resources

Resources

The following list of resources is by no means comprehensive. It is meant simply to get you started on your further inquiry and research on some of the subject matter I present in this book. Like any curious researcher today, you must learn to Google your way to the information you seek.

It is my desire to create a comprehensive resource guide and community connection website that will serve as a research and implementation aid for all parents and practitioners exploring nutrition and dietary information. As this co-creation evolves, please feel free to contact me to participate.

Diets – Community Support
- Nourishing Hope for Autism Diet Community: http://www.facebook.com/group.php?gid=51745596033

GFCF
Books
- *Special Diets for Special Kids* by Lisa Lewis
- *Special Diets for Special Kids 2* by Lisa Lewis
- *Unraveling the Mystery of Autism* by Karen Seroussi
- *Special Eats: Gluten Free & Dairy Free Cooking* by Sueson Vess
- *The Kid-Friendly ADHD and Autism Cookbook* by Dana Laake and Pamela Compart
- *Special Diet Solutions* by Carol Fenster, Ph.D.

Websites
- www.gfcfdiet.com
- www.autismndi.com - Autism Network for Dietary Intervention
- www.autismdiet.com
- www.GFCFmeals.com
- www.celiac (gluten-free only, not casein-free)
- www.enjoylifefoods.com
- www.celiac.org (gluten-free)
- www.glutenfree.com
- www.gluten (gluten-free)
- www.glutenfreeda.com (Gourmet)
- www.glutenfreegourmet.com
- www.glutenfreemall.com (gluten-free)
- www.glutenfreepantry.com
- www.ener-g.com
- www.authenticfoods.com - baking mixes
- www.pamelaproducts.com - cookies and mixes
- gfcf-diet.talkaboutcuringautism.org/substitutions-gfcf-recipes.htm

Yahoo Groups

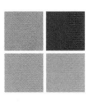

- http://health.groups.yahoo.com/group/GFCFKids/
- http://health.groups.yahoo.com/group/GFCFrecipes/
- http://groups.yahoo.com/group/FOODALLERGYKITCHEN/

SCD

Books and cookbooks
- *Breaking the Vicious Cycle by Elaine Gottschall*
- *Eat Well Feel Well by Kendall Conrad*
- *Healing Foods: Cooking for Celiacs, Colitis, Crohn's and IBS by Sandra Ramacher*

Websites
- www.breakingtheviciouscycle.info
- www.scdiet.com
- www.pecanbread.com
- www.lucyskitchenshop.com
- www.DigestiveWellness.com

Yahoo Groups
- http://health.groups.yahoo.com/group/ElainesChildren/
- http://health.groups.yahoo.com/group/pecanbread/
- http://health.groups.yahoo.com/group/SCDietkids/

Feingold Diet
- Why Can't My Child Behave? By Jane Hersey.
- www.feingold.org
- http://users.bigpond.net.au/allergydietitian/fi/salicylates-list.html - Full list of salicylate-levels in foods
- http://salicylatesensitivity.com
- http://salicylate-sensitivity.allergyanswers.net/

Low Oxalate Diet
- LowOxalate.info
- *The Low Oxalate Cookbook* available at the Vulvar Pain Foundation http://www.vulvarpainfoundation.org/vpfcookbook.htm
- VulvarPainFoundation.org – not autism specific but great research on oxalates
- http://health.groups.yahoo.com/group/Trying_Low_Oxalates/
- Coconut Flour recipes - *Cooking with Coconut Flour* by Bruce Fife

Traditional Diets/Progressive Nutrition (raw dairy, fermented foods)
- *Nourishing Traditions* by Sally Fallon
- *The Fourfold Path to Healing*, by Thomas Cowan, MD
- Weston A. Price Foundation: www.WestonAPrice.org

Resources

- www.mercola.com - Dr. Joseph Mercola.
- www.realmilk.com
- http://health.groups.yahoo.com/group/FailsafeNT/
- http://health.groups.yahoo.com/group/lectins_in_autism/
- http://health.groups.yahoo.com/group/GFCFNN/

Yeast Diets
- *Body Ecology Diet,* by Donna Gates at www.bodyecologydiet.com
- *Feast Without Yeast,* By Bruce Semon
- *The Yeast Connection,* by William Crook

Food Allergies and Sensitivities
- *Is This Your Child? Discovering and Treating Unrecognized Allergies in Children and Adults* by Doris Rapp
- Bioset - http://www.bioset.net
- NAET - http://www.naet.com

Supplements/Products
- Brain Child Nutritionals: www.brainchildnutritionals.com
- Houston Nutraceuticals: www.houstonni.com
- New Beginnings Nutritionals: www.nbnus.com
- Kirkman: www.kirkmanlabs.com
- Klaire Labs: www.klaire.com
- Custom Probiotics: www.customprobiotics.com
- Enzymedica: www.enzymedica.com
- GI ProHealth (GI ProStart Yogurt starter): www.giprohealth.com
- Nordic Naturals: www.nordicnaturals.com
- Nutricia (Neocate and EO28 Splash): www.nutricia.com/
- Celtic Sea Salt: www.celticseasalt.com
- Himalayan Crystal Salt: www.americanbluegreen.com
- Yogurt starter (casein-free): GI ProStart from giprohealth.com or CulturAid by Klaire Labs
- Kefir starter: BodyEcology.com
- Fermentation cultures (kefir grains, kombucha mother): GemCultures.com
- Chocolate Chips (GFCF and soy-free) by Enjoy Life Foods
- Sunflower Seed Butter by Sunbutter
- Coconut products: WildernessFamilyNaturals.com
- Breads From Anna: www.breadsfromanna.com
- Whole Foods Market: www.wholefoods.com
- Nutricia North America: www.nutricia-na.com/
- Bob's Red Mill: www.BobsRedMill.com
- OnlyOats.com
- GlutenfreeOats.com

Visit NourishingHope.com to share
your diet stories and experience.

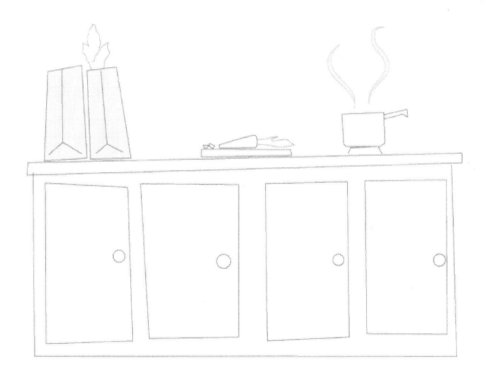

Cooking To Heal
What Parents Are Learning…

"When I first started this journey with my son there was no one out there to help answer my questions on what to cook and how to cook, I felt so alone. I wish I met you then, it would have been much more achievable." - Mom

"This class is one of a kind not to be missed! It is easily accessible, well-organized with clear written guides and tastes that motivate behavior changes." - Mary I.

"Your format is easy to understand, easy to implement and your nutritional knowledge and dedication provided me the encouragement I need - the explanations saved me weeks of trial and error. Thank you!" - Melinda J.

"I did not know nutritious cooking could be tasty too. I now have the confidence that my son will eat my nutritious food without any problems." - Rose C.

"It opened my eyes in how to cook without grains and carbohydrates." - Suzi G,

"I wish all my families of children with an autism spectrum disorder and food reactions could attend Julie's course." Toril H. Jelter MD FAAP

"This class has helped me to understand how to make fermented foods as well as yoghurt. I did not realize how important and also easy to make they are. A little learning can really improve your health." - Welch Family

"Julie serves as an invaluable coach, guiding the viewer through the steps of food prep and an understanding of of exactly how it affects us. I recommend it to my clients as one of the most groundbreaking tools for use in their endeavor. Truly worth owning." Kathleen Reily